An Easy Way To Understand
Vitamins, Minerals & Herbs
Also Included:
Essential Fatty Acids
Enzymes & Amino Acids

Brian B Jacques.

Wisdom For Life Media

"Education is the kindling of a flame, not the filling of a vessel."—Socrates

Publisher: Wisdom For Life Media

While they have made every effort to verify the information provided in this book, neither the author nor the publisher assumes any responsibility for errors in, omissions from, or different interpretation of the subject matter.

The information herein may be subject to varying laws, regulations, and practices in different areas, states and countries. The purchaser or reader assumes all responsibility for use of the information.

All information included within this book is for educational purposes only. The author and publishers do not attempt to diagnose or treat any medical conditions, be it to do with health, diet or exercise.

If you consider that you have any kind of medical condition, then, you should consult a qualified medical practitioner or doctor before starting any vitamin and/or mineral program or supplement regime, exercise or health training program or diet suggested in this book.

This book is not intended for anyone under the age of 18 years, nor is it intended for breast feeding or pregnant women, underweight people or anyone with eating disorders or a health condition that requires special diets or medical treatment.

The author and publishers disclaim any liability for any loss however caused by anyone using the information contained in this book.

ISBN - 13: 978-1500594992

ISBN - 10: 1500594997

Printed and published in the United States of America

Contents

6   Brian B Jacques.

Why Are Vitamins and Minerals So Important?

Vitamins and minerals are as vital in keeping the body going as the fuel, lubricating oil and water in our cars. Without them, we'd simply stop functioning. But how vital are they? Do most of us get the right ones in the right quantities? Let's take a look.

There's been a debate raging for years about whether a proper balanced diet gives you all that you need in terms of vitamins and minerals or whether you need to take supplements to top up your levels. Some doctors are convinced that if you eat properly there's no need for you to take vitamin and mineral supplements, although often they're important for people who are ill, or pregnant women. Others disagree, saying that supplements are essential to make sure we're properly nourished.

So, what is a balanced diet? And is it suitable for everyone? The answer is no, it is not. The human body is made up of approximately 63 percent water, 22 percent protein, 13 percent fat, and 2 percent vitamins and minerals. Everything—every molecule comes from the food you eat and the water you drink.

Someone who is elderly needs a totally different diet to say a top flight sportsman who needs extra amounts of energy to keep his body in peak condition. Likewise, someone who has a physically demanding job would need different dietary requirements to say someone who leads a sedentary lifestyle.

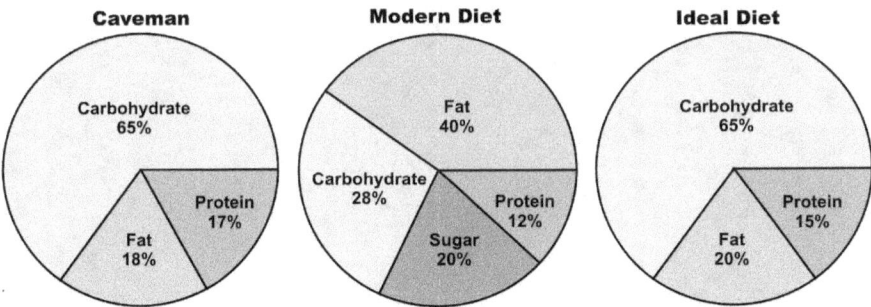

Looking at the pie charts, you will see that the average diet is nothing like it used to be centuries ago. It has shifted, particularly in the past forty years or so to a more high (saturated) fat and sugar diet. A lot of this has come about through clever marketing and the "now society" in which we live, where everything has to be quick and easy. And everything is done on the run, with no time to sit down and eat a meal properly. How often do you see people at lunchtime, walking down the street eating their lunch as they walk, or ordering their lunch at a drive thru facility in a fast food outlet, then the lunch is eaten as the person drives along. This practice is hardly conducive to good digestion and good health.

It is important to eat the best quality food that you can afford, in the correct quantities in order to get the maximum energy, health and freedom from disease. But when we look at the "best quality food", we have to take into account the growing methods of crops, where chemical fertilizers and pesticides are the norm and animal husbandry, where the use of antibiotics and growth promoters are used extensively. All these factors have dramatically changed the quality of our food over the years.

In years gone by, it was common practice for a farmer to exercise crop rotation, and to let certain fields lie fallow for a season in order for them to rest and regenerate themselves. Not anymore! Now as soon as one crop is harvested, the field is plowed over again, it is them treated with chemical pest control agents and nutrients and a new crop is sown.

Many people, of course, eat properly and take the occasional supplement as well, particularly if they've been ill or under the weather. If you do take supplements, make sure you're well informed about exactly what they do, and only take natural ones—not synthetic ones.

We will look at why vitamins and minerals are vital for good health and whether we can benefit from a few extra ones later in this book.

The RDAs

What are RDAs and what do they do? RDA stands for Recommended Dietary Allowance. They are the RDAs of various vitamins and minerals which are set by governments to prevent such diseases as scurvy; they are not designed to ensure good health.

If you look at the RDAs for various countries, you will see that the recommendations vary wildly. And that is not all. The RDAs do not take into account personal factors such as whether a person smokes, drinks alcohol, lives in a polluted environment, is on the pill, or premenstrual, does a lot of exercise or is under a lot of stress.

Tests have been done by researchers on many adults and the result has been that a high percentage of the participants were lacking in the B vitamins.

As an example, the RDA for vitamin C is set at 80mg for the UK and 90mg for the USA. Yet participants in a research project who took over 400mg of vitamin C per day had fewer incidences of colds. This level of vitamin C is way above the RDA for this vitamin.

Not all nutrients have an RDA. Those that do are on the following table, as well as some of those that don't. The table shows the RDA for the United Kingdom (UK) and the United States (USA). By reviewing the table you will see how the recommendations vary.

Nutrient	RDA UK	RDA USA
Vitamin A (mcg)	800	900
Vitamin B1 (mg)	1.1	1.2
Vitamin B2 (mg)	1.4	1.3
Vitamin B3 (mg)	16	16
Vitamin B5 (mg)	6	5
Vitamin B6 (mg)	1.4	1.3
Vitamin B7 (mcg)	50	30
Vitamin B9 (mcg)	200	400
Vitamin B12 (mcg)	2.5	2.4
Vitamin C (mg)	80	90
Vitamin D (mcg)	5	15
Vitamin E (mg)	12	15
Vitamin K (mcg)	75	120

Nutrient	RDA UK	RDA USA
Biotin (mcg)	50	30
Potassium (mg)	2000	4700
Chloride (mg)	800	2300
Choline (mg)	*	550
Omega 3 EPA	*	*
Omega 6 GLA	*	*
Calcium (mg)	800	1000
Chromium (mcg)	40	35
Iodine (mcg)	150	150
Iron (mg)	14	8
Magnesium (mg)	375	400
Manganese (mg)	2	2.3
Selenium (mcg)	55	55
Zinc (mg)	10	11
Phosphorus ((mg)	700	700
Copper (mg)	1	900 (mcg)
Flouride (mg)	3.5	10
Molybdenum (mcg)	50	45
Sodium (mg)	800	1500

* = No RDA

Vitamins for Vitality

So what exactly are vitamins? They each play their own part. They turn on enzymes which are the "spark plugs" that make body functions operate effectively. Vitamins A, C and E are antioxidants which help to neutralize the effects of free radicals in the body. For example, vitamin A from carrots is important for vision and is important for cancer prevention. The B vitamins found in green leafy vegetables help in protein utilization and energy. Vitamin C from such things as oranges helps our bodies to heal when we get a cut, as a protector against the common cold, and as a strengthener of bones and teeth. And vitamin D in milk helps strengthen our bones. We'll have a look in more detail at some of these later.

There are two basic types of vitamin:

Fat soluble. These are stored in the body's fatty tissue and the liver. They reside in your body until they're needed—some for a few days and some for up to six months. Then special carriers take them to wherever they are needed. Vitamins A, D, E and K are all fat soluble.

Water soluble. These are different. When they are water-based they don't tend to get stored in your body as much but travel around in the blood stream. If they are not needed, then, they are expelled in the urine. That means they need to be replaced frequently. These vitamins include vitamin C and the big group of B vitamins—B1 (thiamine), B2 (riboflavin), B3 (niacin), B5 (pantothenic acid), B6 (pyridoxine), B7 (biotin), B9 (folic acid) and B12 (cyanocobalamin), B vitamins are especially important because they not only produce energy but also red blood cells which carry oxygen around your body.

We'll now have a look at each of the vitamins to see exactly why they're important, where they're to be found and the quantities you need to take to preserve your health. I have included the various food sources where each vitamin and mineral is found. However, you can always take a vitamin and / or mineral supplement to rectify any dietary shortfall if required.

Vitamin A

Comes in two forms: the animal form called retinol is found in meat, fish, eggs and dairy products, and its precursor—beta carotene which is found in yellow, red, and orange fruit and vegetables. While high levels of vitamin A can be toxic, this is not the case with beta carotene, which the body converts to vitamin A as it is needed. The residue passes out of the body in the urine. Vitamin A is important in maintaining the health of your skin and mucus membranes in places like the nose. It helps strengthen your immune system to help you recover from infections and assists your night vision.

It's found in foods like liver, oily fish such as mackerel, eggs, fortified milk, margarine, butter, cheese, yogurt, carrots, spinach, broccoli, squash, kale and sweet potatoes.

The (RDA): 900mcg (USA) 800mcg (UK).

Vitamin B1 (Thiamine)

Thiamine works with other B vitamins to break down food. It also keeps our nerves and muscles in good shape. It is important for maintaining energy levels, for brain function and for good digestion. In addition it assists the body to utilize protein.

We find it in pork, vegetables, milk, cheese, peas, fresh and dried fruit, eggs, wholegrain breads and some breakfast cereals.

The (RDA): 1.2mg (USA) 1.1mg (UK).

Vitamin B2 (Riboflavin)

Riboflavin helps maintain the skin, mucous membranes, eyes and the nervous system. It assists in producing steroids and red blood cells and helps the body to absorb iron from food.

You find it in many foods including milk, eggs, breakfast cereals, mushrooms and rice. Riboflavin can be destroyed by ultra violet light so these foods should be kept out of direct sunlight.

The (RDA): 1.3mg (USA) 1.4mg (UK).

Vitamin B3 (Niacin)

Niacin like other vitamins helps convert proteins, fats and carbohydrates into energy as well as keeping the digestive and nervous system healthy. It also helps in balancing blood sugar as well as lowering cholesterol levels. There are two types—nicotinic acid and nicotinamide. They're water soluble so you need them every day.

You get niacin in beef, pork, chicken, wheat flour, maize flour, milk and eggs.

The (RDA): 16mg (USA) 16mg (UK).

Vitamin B5 (Pantothenic Acid)

Pantothenic acid also helps release the energy from food. It is also used by the adrenal glands to produce stress hormones during periods of physical and psychological stress.

You find it in most meat and vegetables especially chicken, beef, potatoes, porridge oats, tomatoes, kidney, eggs, broccoli, whole grains and rice. Some breakfast cereals are fortified with it.

The (RDA): 5mg (USA) 6mg (UK).

Vitamin B6 (Pyridoxine)

Pyridoxine is necessary for metabolizing the amino acids in proteins, the formation of antibodies and red blood cells, and for maintaining a healthy digestive and nervous system.

You find B6 in pork, turkey, chicken, bread, cod and whole cereals such as wheat germ, oatmeal and rice. It's also contained in milk, vegetables, eggs, soy milk, peanuts, potatoes and some breakfast cereals.

The (RDA): 1.3mg (USA) 1.4mg (UK).

Vitamin B7 (Biotin)

Biotin is very important in childhood. It helps your body utilize essential fats and is also important for healthy hair, skin and nails. It also helps turn food into energy as well as being involved in amino acid metabolism. Since its water soluble you need it in your daily diet because it can't be stored.

It's found in a great many foods including kidney, egg yolk and some fruits and vegetables, whole grains, and dried mixed fruit.

The (RDA): 30mcg (USA) 50mcg (UK).

Vitamin B9 (Folic Acid)

Known as folate in its natural form, it works with B12 to form healthy blood cells and helps reduce the risk of defects in babies such as spina bifida.

Folate is found in small amounts in numerous foods but rich sources are breakfast cereals, some types of bread and fruits such as oranges and bananas. It's also found in broccoli, Brussels sprouts, asparagus, peas, rice and chickpeas.

The (RDA): 400mcg (USA) 200mcg (UK).

Vitamin B12 (Cyanocobalamin)

Vitamin B12 helps make red blood cells and generally keeps the nervous system in optimum condition. It helps release energy from the food we eat and it also helps process B9 (folic acid). It deals with the effects of tobacco smoke as well as other toxins in the body. If you don't get enough, you'll probably find that you're anemic. A long term deficiency of B12 can lead to damage of the nervous system. As we get older it becomes more difficult for us to absorb B12.

It's found in fish, meat, poultry and dairy foods. Since you don't get it in vegetables, fruit or grains, vegans or vegetarians may find themselves deficient in it.

The (RDA): 2.4mcg (USA) 2.5mcg (UK).

Note. All the B vitamins work together. If you are taking vitamin B supplements, it is best to take a Balanced B Complex supplement, that way you can be sure that you are getting your B vitamins in the correct ratios.

If you need more of a particular B vitamin, then you can take this in addition to the Balanced B Complex supplement. As always, make sure that whatever supplement you take it is from a natural source—not synthetic.

Vitamin C

This is the one everyone has heard about. It helps protect your body cells and keeps them healthy as well as helping absorb iron from food. It is also used by the adrenal glands to produce hormones and helps to maintain healthy teeth and gums, cartilage, blood vessels and bones.

It is found in fruits such as oranges and kiwi fruit, peppers, broccoli, Brussels sprouts and sweet potatoes.

Compared to other vitamins we need quite a lot every day—minimum 60 mg. However, higher doses are beneficial—up to 2000 mg. It may cause a loose bowel if taken excessively, but this will cease if the dose is reduced. Note! This is not a toxic condition.

The (RDA): 90mg (USA) 80mg (UK).

Vitamin D

Vitamin D helps regulate the amounts of calcium and phosphorous in the body. These substances keep your teeth and bones healthy.

It's only found in a small number of foods such as liver, oily fish and egg yolk. Other sources include margarine, cheese, butter, breakfast cereals and fortified milk. Most of the vitamin D we get is made in the skin because of its reaction to sunlight. Incidentally, most people—and especially children—lack vitamin D either through a lack of sun exposure, or it is lacking in the diet.

In children, vitamin D is important for proper growth and development. It is also important for the synthesis of calcium. If you're pregnant or breast-feeding you should supplement with vitamin D. Older people especially should take a vitamin D supplement. You should also take it if you eat no meat or oily fish, rarely go outdoors or cover up when you do.

The (RDA): 15mcg (USA) 5mcg (UK).

Vitamin E

Vitamin E is a fat soluble vitamin which is needed to help maintain a lot of the tissues in your body especially the eyes, skin and liver. As it is an antioxidant vitamin, it stops your lungs getting damaged by polluted air and it also helps the production of red blood cells.

The richest sources of vitamin E are from plant oils such as soy, corn and olive oil as well as seeds, nuts, wheat germ, green leafy vegetables, egg yolk and olives.

The (RDA): 15mg (USA) 12mg (UK).

Vitamin K (Phylloquinone)

Vitamin K is important in blood clotting to ensure that wounds heal properly; it's also needed to build strong bones.

Spinach, cereals, vegetable oils and broccoli are especially rich in it. You get small amounts in meats like pork and dairy produce such as cheese. But you also produce it yourself—in the friendly bacteria in your intestines.

The (RDA): 120mcg (USA) 75mcg (UK).

Beta-carotene

An antioxidant vitamin. The antioxidant content gives orange and yellow fruits their color. Beta-carotene is turned into vitamin A in the body.

It's found in green and leafy vegetables such as spinach, carrots, red peppers and fruits such as melon, mango and apricots.

It is non-toxic in high doses as any excess passes out in the urine.

The (RDA): N/A (USA) 800mcg (UK).

Co-enzyme Q10 (Co-Q10)

Co-enzyme Q10 (Co-Q10) is an antioxidant substance similar to a vitamin. It is manufactured in the body and is found in all body cells. Cells use it to provide energy that your body needs for cell growth and maintenance.

As a person ages, the production of Co-Q10 declines. Additionally certain medication—statins taken to lower cholesterol in particular, destroy Co-Q10. It is therefore beneficial to take a Co-Q10 supplement to make up for the shortfall.

Small amounts are found in many different foods. However, the highest concentration is found in organ meats: heart, liver and kidneys. It is also found in oily fish such as sardines and mackerel as well as peanuts and soy oil.

Co-Q10 has been used for many years by people with various cardiovascular conditions with positive results.

There is no (RDA) for Co-Q10.

The Magic of Minerals

Every time you move your arms, blink your eyes turn your head—you are using minerals. Minerals are not produced by the body you get them from your food; therefore minerals are important for almost every body function. Calcium, magnesium and phosphorus are essential for bones and teeth. Nerve transmissions essential for brain and muscle actions depend on calcium, magnesium, sodium and potassium. Chromium is essential for controlling blood sugar levels. Zinc—an antioxidant mineral is essential as a free radical scavenger, also for body development as well as repair and renewal. Zinc and selenium—another antioxidant mineral supports your immune system.

There are two types of minerals—macro or essential minerals, and trace minerals which are needed in very tiny amounts by the body.

As mentioned above, they have three main functions:

- Building strong bones and teeth
- Controlling body fluids inside and outside cells
- Converting the food we eat into energy

The main macro or essential minerals are:

- Calcium
- Iron
- Magnesium
- Phosphorus
- Potassium
- Sodium
- Sulfur

The trace elements are:

- Boron
- Cobalt
- Copper
- Chromium
- Germanium
- Iodine
- Manganese

- Molybdenum

- Selenium

- Silicon

- Zinc

Let's have a look in more detail at the important things that minerals and trace elements do in the body.

Boron

This trace element assists the body in making the best use of fats, glucose, estrogen and other minerals such as copper, calcium and magnesium. It occurs widely in plants, oceans, rocks and soil and can be found in green vegetables, fruit and nuts.

There is no (RDA) for Boron.

Calcium

Calcium is one of the most crucial minerals we need. As well as building strong teeth and bones, it's important in regulating muscle contractions which includes the heart beat. It also ensures that your blood clots normally when you receive a cut. It is also an important mineral for maintaining the correct acid / alkaline balance

The main sources of calcium are milk, cheese and dairy products as well as green leafy vegetables such as cabbage broccoli, and okra (ladies' fingers). You also find it in soy beans, tofu, nuts, and bread made with fortified flour and fish such as sardines and pilchards when you eat the bones.

When taking calcium as a supplement, it is preferable to take it in a combination form of calcium and magnesium. Vitamin D should also be in the formula as it helps with the absorption of calcium. Also important is phosphorus, which works with calcium, boron, copper, and zinc (an antioxidant mineral).

Calcium supplements on their own can cause constipation in some people. Magnesium helps to counteract the constipation effect of the calcium. As separate supplements, take roughly half the amount of magnesium to what you are taking of calcium.

The (RDA): 1000mg (USA) 800mg (UK).

Coral Calcium

Elsewhere in this book I have mentioned how the Western diet is acid forming which can lead to a condition called acidosis. Well, coral calcium is naturally alkaline, so it can be really important for those people who want to keep their pH levels within the normal range. Coral Calcium is especially important for females as it helps support mineral levels in the female body, especially in regard to natural hormone fluctuations.

As well as supplying important calcium to the body, any formulation should also contain magnesium as these two minerals help each other. Vitamin D should be in the formula too as it aids in the absorption of calcium.

Middle-aged women as well as elderly men and women and those persons with a family history of osteoporosis, and white and Asian women between the ages of 11–35 can really benefit from an adequate calcium supplementation program.

There is no (RDA) for Coral Calcium.

Chromium

Chromium helps to regulate insulin in the body and therefore has an effect on how much energy you get from your food. It helps to reduce food cravings and improves lifespan. It is also important for proper heart function.

This trace element can be found in soil, air, water, animals and plants. In food you get it from meat, whole grains, spices and lentils.

The (RDA): 35mcg (USA) 40mcg (UK).

Cobalt

Cobalt forms part of the structure of vitamin B12 which I discussed earlier. It's found widely in the environment. Fish, nuts, leafy green vegetables such as spinach, broccoli and cereals containing oats are all good food sources.

Basically, to get enough cobalt you need to make sure you get enough vitamin B12.

There is no (RDA) for Cobalt.

Copper

Copper is important in the production of both red and white blood cells. It also causes the release of iron to form hemoglobin, which is an iron-containing protein attached to red blood cells. This transports oxygen from the lungs to the rest of the body. Hemoglobin binds with oxygen in the lungs, which it then exchanges for carbon dioxide at the cellular level. It then transports the carbon dioxide back to the lungs to be exhaled.

Copper helps in child growth, the development of the brain and nervous system and producing strong bones. In addition, it assists in maintaining healthy skin and hair color and is also used to diminish the effects of rheumatoid arthritis related inflammation.

It's found in nuts, shellfish and meat offal.

The (RDA): 900mcg (USA) 1mg (UK).

Germanium

Many of the important herbs and medicinal plants traditionally used in healing, including ginseng, garlic, comfrey, and aloe vera, all contain substantial amounts of germanium. The therapeutic benefits of these herbs may be linked to the high amounts of germanium they contain.

Germanium also has antioxidant potential, and provides energy from carbohydrates in the diet. It's also found in a wide range of foods including beans, tomato juice, oysters and tuna, as well as those sources mentioned above.

Germanium comes in two forms—organic and inorganic. Inorganic germanium supplements have been withdrawn from sale because in this form they can damage the nervous system, liver and kidneys. The best organic supplements traditionally come from Japan where much of the research work has been done, particularly as a cancer preventative.

There is no (RDA) for Germanium.

Iodine

Iodine helps make thyroid hormones which keep cells healthy and regulate your body's metabolic rate. It's found in seawater, seaweed, Black Walnut, rocks and soil as well as cow's milk. Fish and shellfish are especially rich in it. But it's also found in plant foods such as cereals and grains but this depends to a large extent on the amount of iodine found in the soils where those plants are grown.

Every cell in the body needs iodine. Interestingly, if you put a small amount of this brown liquid on the back of your hand it will have disappeared within 24 hours. In fact it will have been absorbed by the body's cells which "line up" to get a "fix" of this important mineral.

Inflammation is one of the greatest threats to the human body. And is often a precursor to more serious health conditions developing. Iodine is very effective in reducing inflammation in the body and thus helping to protect you.

The (RDA): 150mcg (USA) 150mcg (UK).

Iron

This is another of those essential minerals just about everyone has heard of. It's vital in the production of red blood cells to move oxygen around the body. The traditional way to get iron into your system was through organ meat such as liver. But there are plenty of other sources such as beans, nuts, dried fruit, whole grains, breakfast cereals, soybean flour and most green leafed vegetables like water cress and curly kale.

A lot of people think that spinach is a good source but the problem is that spinach contains a substance which makes it harder for the body to absorb the iron from it. Strangely enough, both tea and coffee also contain substances which bind together with iron and make it more difficult for it to be absorbed. So cutting down on tea and coffee could boost your iron levels—and reduce your caffeine intake too.

On the other hand, eating foods rich in vitamin C at the same time as foods containing iron from non-meat sources might actually help with iron absorption. So fruit juice with your breakfast cereal or beans might prove beneficial.

Women who lose a lot of blood during their menstrual cycle may need iron supplements.

Women need more iron than men—around 14.8 mg as opposed to 8.7 mg for men.

The (RDA): 8mg (USA) 14mg (UK).

Magnesium

Magnesium helps convert food to energy and makes sure that the parathyroid glands (which produce hormones to promote bone health) are working normally. It is also important for bones and teeth, as well as for the heart and nervous system. It is important for calcium uptake as well as being an anti-inflammatory mineral.

Magnesium can be obtained from nuts and green leafy vegetables as well as bread, meat, fish and dairy products.

The (RDA): 400mg (USA) 375mg (UK).

Manganese

The trace element manganese helps activate over twenty enzymes in the body which assist in such things as digesting your food. It's often found in supplements. It is also important for healthy bone formation, cartilage, tissues and nerve function.

It occurs in bread, nuts, cereals and green vegetables such as peas and runner beans. Perhaps its main source for a lot of people is tea, drunk without milk.

The (RDA): 2.3mg (USA) 2mg (UK).

Molybdenum

This is actually a heavy metal but as a trace element it's vital in activating those enzymes which produce and repair genetic material. It helps purge the body of waste protein by-products as well as detoxifying the body of free radicals, petroleum by-products and sulphites.

It is found in a lot of food, especially those vegetables which grow above ground such as peas, broccoli, spinach and cauliflower. It also occurs in nuts, tinned vegetables and oats.

The (RDA): 45mcg (USA) 50mcg (UK).

Nickel

Nickel not only regulates the amount of iron in your body but it also plays a role in the production of red blood cells. It's important to note that one in ten people have an allergy to nickel so that if they come into contact with coins or jewelery containing it they may come out in a rash. The same can happen if you take supplements containing nickel and have an allergy.

Nickel is very widespread in the environment and lentils, nuts and oats are good sources.

There is no (RDA) for Nickel.

Phosphorous

Phosphorous has a number of important functions such as building strong bones and teeth and helping to release food energy. It is a component of DNA and RNA, as well as helping to maintain the acid/alkaline balance of your body.

It's found in dairy foods, fish, poultry, bread, rice and oats.

The (RDA): 700mg (USA) 700mg (UK).

Potassium

Potassium controls the balance of fluids in your body and it may also help to reduce blood pressure. Potassium makes it possible for essential nutrients to move into body cells, and for waste products to be eliminated from them. It is also involved in insulin secretion to control blood sugar which supplies energy to the body.

Fruit such as bananas are rich in it as are vegetables, pulses, nuts, seeds, milk, fish, shellfish, beef, chicken, turkey and bread.

The (RDA): 4700mg (USA) 2000mg (UK).

Selenium

Selenium plays a key role in the function of your immune system, in the production of thyroid hormones and in reproduction. It's also a key player in the body's antioxidant defense system which prevents damage to cells and tissue. It is an antioxidant mineral and works with vitamin E.

Brazil nuts, bread, fish, meat and eggs are all rich sources.

The (RDA): 55mcg (USA) 55mcg (UK).

Silicon

More well-known for the chips in our computers and other electrical gadgets, silicon helps maintain strong bones and helps keep your connective tissue healthy.

It is found in grains such as barley, oats and rice as well as in fruit and vegetables.

There is no (RDA) for Silicon.

Sodium chloride

Better known as salt, There has been a lot of discussion in the media and in government concerning the tendency for people to eat too much of it, especially in such things as processed foods, which often have very high levels added. Indeed most people do eat too much. But it's a vital substance in keeping the fluids in the body well balanced. And because it's a central ingredient of the juices in your stomach and intestines it helps you digest the food you eat.

Salt is found in low levels in virtually all foods. On average most people eat around 9.5 grams a day.

The (RDA): 1500mg (USA) 800mg (UK).

Sulfur

Sulfur's functions include the production of tissue such as cartilage. It is involved in many key body functions such as reducing inflammation, pain from arthritis and detoxification.

Sulfur is also a constituent of keratin and collagen which are found in hair, skin and nails. Therefore sulfur compounds are beneficial for these three areas.

One of the best forms of sulfur is the supplement MSM (methyl sulfonyl methane).

The therapeutic dose according to research into pain relief using MSM is a daily concentration between 1,500mg—3,000mg.

There is no (RDA)for Sulfur.

Tin

Very little research has been done on tin and its role in human health. One study showed psychological benefits of decreased depression and fatigue and an increase in positive mood and well being in some study recipients, while others experienced a reduction in headaches, asthma, insomnia and general levels of pain.

Tin is available in small amounts from virtually all fruits and vegetables. It is absorbed by plants from the soil. How much is found in food depends on the levels in the soil where the plants are grown.

There is no (RDA) for Tin.

Vanadium

Some interesting animal studies indicate that vanadium may help to normalize glucose levels, enhance athletic performance, and lower blood pressure. However, beneficial effects have yet to be conclusively proven in human studies.

Vanadium is a trace mineral that is essential for maintaining a healthy body. Vanadium is an opposite of molybdenum, which is another trace mineral, in that it works in tandem with it. Together, the two minerals help keep each other in check and provide several health benefits to humans.

In animal and human studies it has been found that vanadium helped to reduce blood sugar levels and also increased insulin sensitivity in those with type 1 and type 11 diabetes.

Food sources are seafood, cereals, mushrooms, parsley, corn, and soy.

There is no (RDA) for Vanadium.

Zinc

Zinc is an antioxidant mineral that helps make new cells and enzymes. It also functions with vitamins A and E to manufacture thyroid hormones.

It helps to process protein, fat and carbohydrate from foods and also with the healing of wounds.

Zinc is an important mineral in appetite control and a deficiency can cause a loss of taste and smell, thus creating a need for stronger tasting foods (which tend to be sweeter, saltier and more fattening.)

It's found in things like meat, shellfish, milk, dairy foods and cereals.

The (RDA): 11mg (USA) 15mg (UK).

Zinc Lozenges

Zinc is often combined with Echinacea and Licorice Root (as a natural sweetener) to treat the effects of a sore throat or other mouth infections. It also supplies excellent immune system support.

Essential Fatty Acids (EFA's)

Essential Fatty Acids are so called because you have to get them from your diet—the body cannot make them itself. There are two essential fatty acids: omega-3 and omega-6. These two are the building blocks that make the twenty fatty acids that the body needs for good health.

Omega-3 Essential Fatty Acids.

There are several different types of omega-3 essential fatty acids:

Alpha Linolenic Acid (ALA) good sources are: canola, flaxseed, rapeseed, soybeans, and walnuts.

Eicosapentaenoic acid (EPA) which is obtained from cold water, oily fish: herrings, salmon, sardines and tuna are good sources.

Docosahexaenoic acid (DHA) which is also obtained from cold water, oily fish: herrings, salmon, sardines and tuna are good sources.

Omega-6 Essential Fatty Acids

There are several different types of omega-6 essential fatty acids:

Linoleic Acid (LA) good sources are corn oil, cottonseed oil, peanut oil, rice bran oil, safflower oil, Soybean oil and sunflower oil.

Arachidonic acid (AA) obtained from: dairy products, eggs, meat and peanut oil.

Gamma Linolenic Acid (GLA) this is obtained mainly from plant based oils, such as: black currant oil, borage oil, and evening primrose oil. In addition, most of these oils also contain some linoleic acid (LA).

Essential fatty acids are important for the manufacture of cell membranes as well as important hormones and neurotransmitters—chemical substances that pass messages between different cells which tell the body what to do.

They are also involved in the manufacture of prostaglandins in your body. These hormone-like substances help control many different activities. Some of these activities include such things as inflammation, pain, and unbelievably, some cause swelling and some reduce swelling. They are involved in allergic reactions, blood clotting and the manufacture of other hormones.

Prostaglandins also have a role to play in controlling blood pressure, heart and kidney function, body temperature in addition to being involved in the digestive system.

Being natural blood thinners, fatty acids help prevent blood clots, which can trigger a heart attack or stroke.

Arthritis and autoimmune diseases can be relieved by the natural anti-inflammatory compounds found in essential fatty acids.

If you experience skin problems or you have dull or brittle hair, if your nails split easily, or you have dandruff or eczema, then your diet could be lacking in essential fatty acids.

Essential Fatty Acids have an important role to play in good digestive and intestinal systems health. They help maintain cell stability in addition to increasing the thickness of cells lining the intestinal tract, as well as the villi which enhances the absorption of nutrients. All this leads to better digestion and improved health.

DHA—an omega-3 fatty acid is the most plentiful fat in the brain. It is important for ensuring that chemical messages pass effectively between the brain cells. Copious quantities of omega-3 fatty acids are also found in the retina of the eye.

Omega-3 fatty acids are also found in high concentrations in breast milk. Babies require it for their brain growth and vision development.

Low levels of essential fatty acids in the diet have been linked to vision problems, mood swings, memory loss and dementia.

So how much essential fatty acid should you take? It all depends on such factors as: what type of diet you have? The typical Western diet is very rich in omega-6 essential fatty acids which can cause a hormone imbalance leading to various health problems.

The ideal ratio is one portion of omega-3 to 5 portions of omega-6. In the typical Western diet which is high in saturated fat the ratio is often one portion of omega-3 to 20 portions of omega-6. To counteract this imbalance it might be a good idea to use the following formula. For every portion of omega 6, take 2 portions of omega-3. If you find it difficult to achieve this with your diet, then consider taking an omega-3 supplement. Incidentally, there is no Recommended Daily Allowance (RDA) for essential fatty acids. Men may need to take more than women. Also, if a person suffers from stress or health problems then more may be needed.

You may need to do your own experimentation to see how much you need. Have a look at your skin. If it is dry, then you should consider taking more omega-3. Skin that is well supplied with omega-3 feels supple to the touch. Remember in cold weather the skin can dry out necessitating an increased supply of omega-3.

Essential Fatty Acid Supplements

Black Currant Oil

Black currant oil is a rich source of omega-3 (linolenic essential fatty acid (EFA), alpha linolenic acid (ALA), and omega-6 gamma linoleic essential fatty acid (GLA), along with other important polyunsaturated fatty acids.

Fatty acids are involved in most body functions, from maintaining body temperature to providing a cushion for and protecting body tissue as well as protecting the nervous system and creating energy.

Interestingly, before the discovery of the benefits of black currant oil, the only other known sources of GLA were mother's milk and evening primrose oil.

CLA

CLA, or conjugated linoleic acid, is a mixture of essential fatty acids that are important for maintaining healthy body functions.

CLA helps to sustain lean muscle mass as well as enhancing the burning of fat, which makes it a useful product in a weight-loss regime.

DHA

DHA (docosahexaenoic acid) is an omega-3 fatty acid sourced from oily fish such as herring, mackerel, salmon, and sardines that is absorbed into the fatty perimeter of cells where it exerts its biochemical properties. DHA offers many benefits. It supports and protects the nervous system and supports brain and eye health as well as the health of the skin.

Evening Primrose Oil

Evening Primrose is a plant that grows throughout the US and Europe. The plant grows close to the ground and the oil is found in the plants seeds. This oil is rich in gamma linolenic acid (GLA, an omega-6 essential fatty acid).

The oil is traditionally used to treat various skin conditions such as eczema and dermatitis and to alleviate breast tenderness from premenstrual syndrome (PMS).

Evening Primrose Oil seems to be more effective for the above conditions when taken with an omega-3 supplement from fish oil (derived from oily cold water fish such as salmon, tuna, mackerel and sardines) to create a healthy body balance.

Evening Primrose Oil is also used in the manufacture of some cosmetics and soap.

It is available as an oil or in capsule form. It should be kept out of direct sunlight and preferably stored in a refrigerator to prevent rancidity.

Flax Seed Oil

The Flax plant is a blue, flowering plant that is grown in Ireland and the western Canadian prairies. No part of the plant is wasted. The inner stems contain fibers that are made into linen for use in the manufacture of bedding as well as clothes. The oil-rich seeds of the plant, known as flax seed oil or linseed oil, are used for cattle feed, in the paint industry, and as a rich source of omega-3 and -6 essential fatty acids for human consumption. These natural essential fatty acids are used for the general well-being and support of most body systems.

Flax Seed is considered to be one of nature's richest sources of alpha-linolenic acid (ALA)—(an omega-3 fatty acid)—as well as containing omega-6 essential fatty acids. In addition, flax seed oil contains B vitamins, potassium, lecithin, magnesium, fiber, protein, and zinc.

It also contains Lignans which are a type of fiber that is changed by "friendly bacteria" in the gut into compounds that fight against cancer.

Krill Oil

Krill are tiny crustaceans that serve as a good food source for whales, seals, and other ocean mammals. They also provide a rich source of essential omega-3 fatty acids, including EPA and DHA.

Omega-3 essential fatty acids are important for cardiovascular and brain health as well as providing support for joints and the skin. Krill is a natural source of powerful antioxidant carotenoids.

Krill oil naturally contains phospholipids, which attach to omega-3 fatty acids, enhancing their absorption in the body. Phospholipids strengthen cell membranes as well as making them more elastic, which helps to keep toxins out and let nutrients and oxygen in.

Omega-3 Essential Fatty Acids

There are several different types of omega-3 essential fatty acids:

Alpha Linolenic Acid (ALA) good sources are: canola, flaxseed, rapeseed, soybeans, and walnuts.

Eicosapentaenoic acid (EPA) which is obtained from cold water, oily fish: herrings, salmon, sardines and tuna are good sources.

Docosahexaenoic acid (DHA) which is also obtained from cold water, oily fish: herrings, salmon, sardines and tuna are good sources.

Not a Vitamin, Not a Mineral, Not a Herb

Acai Berry

The acai berry is an inch-long reddish, purple fruit. It comes from the acai palm tree which is native to the Brazilian Rainforest.

Acai Berry is a very powerful antioxidant which contains both anthocyanins and flavonoids.

The word anthocyanin comes from two Greek words meaning "plant" and "blue." Anthocyanins provide the red, purple and blue color in fruits, vegetables, and flowers. Foods that are strongly colored such as acai, blueberries, red grapes and red wine, have very high anthocyanin activity.

Because of its high antioxidant activity, the acai berry is very effective at neutralizing the effects of free radical damage.

Currently there is a lot of marketing hype around acai berry with various claims of what it can do. It is heavily marketed for weight loss and is often combined with other herbal ingredients to make a combination product to treat various conditions in the human body. It is also marketed as an antioxidant to fight free radical damage.

In its native form, the fruit spoils very easily, so it is not available in your local supermarket, health food store, or on the Internet. However, it is often freeze dried for later use. This drying process does not appear to reduce the effectiveness of the fruit.

Acai oil is also used in some beauty and cosmetic products because of its high antioxidant activity. What makes it so useful for the cosmetics industry is that when it is processed and stored for long periods of time, the antioxidant potency does not degrade with age.

Acai oil is used in some facial and body creams, anti-aging skin treatments, shampoos and conditioners.

For human consumption it is available as a capsule or in liquid form.

Activated Charcoal

Charcoal is highly absorbent. Activated Charcoal can help in cases of poisoning or severe diarrhea as it absorbs irritants and toxins in the digestive tract. It may also help lower cholesterol levels as well as relieving the effects of foul belching and severe smelly gas. An alternative to activated charcoal is to use bentonite clay.

Alpha Lipoic Acid

Alpha lipoic acid is a very powerful antioxidant fatty acid which is found in every cell of the body. The body utilizes it to convert glucose (blood sugar) into energy for normal body functions.

Alpha lipoic acid is able to function in both water and fat, unlike the more common antioxidants vitamins C which functions in water and vitamin E which functions in fat.

A unique feature of Alpha Lipoic Acid is that it can recycle antioxidants such as vitamin C and glutathione after they have been expended. Meaning, they can be used again to fulfill body functions. Glutathione is an important antioxidant that assists the body in eliminating harmful substances. Alpha lipoic acid enhances the formation of glutathione.

Although the body manufactures Alpha Lipoic Acid, it is also found in brewer's yeast, broccoli, Brussels sprouts, organ meats, peas, rice bran and spinach.

Alpha Lipoic Acid is also intimately involved in brain function by crossing the blood brain barrier (a wall of structural cells and tiny blood vessels) to protect nerve and brain tissue from the effects of free radical damage.

Other uses for Alpha Lipoic Acid include: supporting the body after chemotherapy, dietary deficiencies, alcoholism, diabetes, kidney disease, Lyme disease, shingles and thyroid disorders.

Alpha Lipoic Acid is available as a supplement in capsule form, and in studies the daily amount that was best tolerated by the body, and to supply adequate amounts was 600mg, taken on an empty stomach.

Apple Cider Vinegar

Excellent for vaginal yeast infections and external candida conditions, it has good anti-fungal properties and can be added to warm bath water enabling a person to soak in it.

Bentonite (montmorillonite) Clay

Bentonite clay is very quick acting as it has the ability to bind the stools together. It does this by binding irritants in the gastrointestinal tract. One option is to combine the bentonite clay with a small quantity of applesauce to make the clay more palatable. Applesauce contains pectin—another binding agent. Incidentally pectin is also used in jam making to make the fruit "set".

Chinese Red Yeast Rice

Chinese Red Yeast Rice was first documented by the Tang Dynasty in 800AD. It is part of the daily diet of Chinese, Japanese and Asian communities to this day. Traditionally it is used as a food preservative, food colorant (it is responsible for the red color of Peking duck), as a spice, and an ingredient in rice wine.

Historical Medicinal uses include: a treatment for improving blood circulation, alleviating indigestion and diarrhea. In more recent time it has been used very effectively to lower cholesterol levels. This is due to it containing a family of monacolins (polyketides) with the ability to inhibit cholesterol synthesis and lower plasma cholesterol levels.

Traditionally the method used to make red yeast rice is to ferment the yeast naturally on a bed of non-glutinous whole rice kernels. This is rather a slow process which has been mechanized to produce dietary supplements containing the rice, yeast and Monascus fungus which is all contained in a gelatin capsule.

There are a number of natural compounds in Chinese Red Yeast Rice including: fatty acids and pigments in addition to monacolins (polyketides) mentioned above. The monacolins are believed to be the main component of the yeast's cholesterol lowering activity.

When combined with diet and lifestyle changes, Chinese Red Yeast Rice could be a good choice to lower cholesterol without side effects.

Colloidal Silver

Colloidal silver has numerous uses and has been found to be effective against many surface and internal micro-organisms, viruses, protozoa, amoeba, fungi, parasites and yeasts. It works by in-activating the enzyme that is responsible for the multiplication of many of these invaders.

There are many different colloidal silver products on the market. You need to source one that contains 99.9 percent pure silver, without any additives, apart from water.

Hoodia Gordonii

Hoodia is actually a succulent plant that grows in the semi-deserts of South Africa, Botswana, Namibia, and Angola. It grows in clumps of green upright stems which after five years produce a pale purple flower, at which time the plant can be harvested.

Interestingly, there are said to be more than 13 varieties of hoodia. But only hoodia gordonii has so far been identified as containing an active ingredient, a steroidal glycoside that has been named "p57".

Much of the marketing hype stems from stories of San Bushmen who live in the Kalahari Desert. These bushmen have taken hoodia for thousands of years to stave off hunger pangs and thirst whilst on long hunting trips. Today hoodia gordonii is sold as a weight loss product and is available as a capsule, powder, and tea or liquid.

Lecithin

Lecithin is found in many food sources including cabbage, cauliflower, eggs, garbanzo beans, organic meat, seeds, soy beans, split peas and nuts. It is also manufactured by the body provided the correct nutrients are available for it to do so. Unfortunately this is not always the case with the average Western diet; therefore supplementation is almost always necessary. Supplements can be in either liquid or capsule form. Lecithin is non-toxic.

Lecithin is an important phospholipid which is needed and utilized by all body cells as well as the heart, liver and kidneys. As it is a fat itself, it adheres to cell and nerve linings, forming a slippery barrier to prevent cholesterol and other fats from sticking. This ensures that blood flows more freely.

When Lecithin breaks down body fats, it then transports these fats to the liver and helps convert them into usable energy.

Methyl Sulfonyl Methane (MSM)

Methyl Sulfonyl Methane is a sulfur dietary supplement that starts life in the sea. Plankton in the sea release sulfur compounds which rise into the atmosphere where ultra violet light converts them into MSM and DMSO (dimethyl sulfoxide)—a precursor to MSM.

MSM and DMSO return to earth attached to rain droplets. MSM is found in grains, vegetables, fruits, meat and poultry.

MSM is an organic form of sulfur that is found in living tissues. MSM is the only dietary supplement that relieves allergies and arthritic conditions at the same time. In the structural system it is an excellent treatment for arthritis, muscle pains and bursitis. Additionally, it supports connective tissue such as ligaments, tendons, and muscle.

Sulfur is an important element in maintaining good health. But it is lacking in the Western diet. Therefore it would be worth considering as a preventative product.

Morinda Citrifolia (Noni)

A native of the Polynesian Islands—Tahiti and Hawaii—Morinda Citrifolia (Noni) has been used by the Polynesians for over 2,000 years in a variety of treatments for various infections including: bacterial, viral, fungal and also for tumors. Additionally it has been used as a hypotensive, for anti-inflammatory conditions, and to support the immune system. Further uses include: boosting metabolism in a weight management program.

Morinda is available in capsules and also as a liquid. In liquid form the raw Morinda has a very bitter taste, so it is often sweetened with natural liquorice or glycerin.

Proanthocyanidins

Often sold under the trade name Pycnogenol. Proanthocyanidins are powerful antioxidants obtained from grape seed and pine bark. They help prevent cell damage by quenching oxidative free radicals. This combination of antioxidant nutrients has been shown to be many times more powerful than vitamin C or E. Proanthocyanidins also improve the integrity of collagen fibers, in addition to strengthening tissues in the skin, blood vessels, muscles, cartilage and other connective tissue areas of the body.

Tea Tree Oil

A native of Australia, Tea Tree Oil has many uses. It is highly prized for its antiseptic and anti-bacterial benefits. It is used to treat acne, athlete's foot, abscesses, boils, dandruff and Pyorrhea. It is also used to sterilize cuts.

Algae and Seaweed:
Chlorella

Chlorella is a single-celled green algae and contains over 19 amino acids. Of these eight are the essential ones in addition to beta carotene (which the body converts to vitamin A as needed). It also contains potassium and other important vitamins and minerals, plus enzymes.

Chlorella has natural antioxidant properties and as such, is a good detoxifier, cell enhancer and blood cleanser.

When taken as a liquid it eliminates body odors from the digestive tract, and is also an excellent mouth wash to eliminate bad breath.

Irish Moss

Irish moss is a type of seaweed that soothes an irritated gastrointestinal tract. It is also used in hand and body lotion products to alleviate various skin conditions.

Kelp

Kelp is a brown algae that comes from the sea. It responds to sunlight and takes in minerals and other nutrients from the water. It is an excellent source of iodine. Iodine is needed for proper functioning of the thyroid and pituitary glands.

The thyroid is responsible for maintaining metabolism and body temperature. In fact during stressful periods, the thyroid can work overtime to try and normalize body functions, therefore supplementing with kelp can be very beneficial for boosting energy.

A proper functioning metabolism is also important for maintaining weight control, which can sometimes be a problem when the body is under stress, and a person is susceptible to "binge eat" on comfort foods.

Spirulina

Spirulina is a type of fresh-water blue-green algae composed of approximately 65-71 percent protein making it one of the richest known sources of vegetable protein. This protein is biologically complete, meaning it contains all 9 essential amino acids in their proper ratios.

Much of the protein in spirulina is in the form of biliprotein which has been pre-digested by the algae itself, making it 5 times easier to break down than either meat or soy protein. In fact, the digestibility of spirulina protein is rated 85 percent, compared to approximately 20 percent for beef protein.

This easy to digest type of protein is especially beneficial for those suffering from problems associated with excessive animal protein and refined foods intake: namely those with arthritis, cancer, diabetes, hypoglycemia, obesity, or similar degenerative conditions.

Friendly Bacteria:

Acidophilus

Provides friendly bacteria which normally resides in the intestines and is often destroyed through taking prescription antibiotics, using the birth pill or steroids. It can also be depleted though a dietary shortfall. These friendly bacteria can be replaced by taking a supplement in capsule form and/or through the diet.

Bifidophilus

A probiotic supplement. Bifidophilus products contain living organisms from various strains of "friendly" bacteria to help replace depleted bacteria in the colon. They are necessary for proper immune function, and to help balance the digestive system.

Probiotics are very beneficial after taking a course of antibiotics. Antibiotics not only kill foreign invaders, but they kill "friendly" bacteria too.

Probiotics

Probiotics are an essential part of good health as they keep "balance" in the body, as well as aiding the digestive, intestinal and immune systems. These "friendly" bacteria produce hydrogen peroxide which kills candida; thus in addition to its other health giving benefits it is a good supplement for anyone suffering from a candida yeast infection.

Fiber:

Psyllium

An excellent source of dietary fiber, psyllium is gluten free and is therefore a useful fiber source for those suffering from celiac disease or a gluten intolerance.

It expands dramatically from the size of the original seeds and it is therefore essential to drink plenty of water with this product. Psyllium absorbs toxins from the intestinal tract and binds them to fecal matter for elimination.

As it is a bulking agent, it often gives a feeling of fullness and discourages a person from over eating. One of the main causes of constipation is a lack of fiber in the diet.

Guar Gum

Is often used in fiber blends as it provides soluble digestible fiber. The body needs non-soluble as well as soluble fiber. Guar gum soaks toxins up like a sponge. It has a laxative effect, curbs appetite and is beneficial in lowering cholesterol.

Supplements, Free Radicals and Antioxidants

At the beginning of this book I discussed a "balanced diet" and "we get everything from our food", as I explained that is not the case. Listening to the so called "experts", they never actually say what a balanced diet is. It is just a sweeping statement that encompasses everyone and everything, when in fact no two people are exactly alike. Everyone has different dietary needs as well as different lifestyles.

In his book *Biochemical Individuality* Dr Roger Williams, who discovered vitamin B5 (pantothenic acid), explains how each person has organs that are different shapes and sizes, how each person has different levels of enzymes and different requirements for vitamins and minerals. A ten fold difference in requirements from one person to another is not unusual. So how come we get everything we need from a balanced diet, without saying what a balanced diet is.

The only light that is shed on the 'balanced diet" is to refer to the basic food groups: grains, dairy products, meat, fish and poultry, fruits and vegetables. However, if you listen to the audio tape *Dead Doctors Don't Lie* by Dr Joel Wallach, he explains how he conducted hundreds of autopsies which revealed that the vast majority of deaths were caused by diseases brought on by nutritional deficiencies.

People tend to eat for taste, not nutrition, and it can be very difficult to change a person's eating habits. It is a fact that junk food tastes good and people will not be told to eat fruit and vegetables. This is one reason why informed people understand the importance of supplementing the modern diet with extra vitamins, minerals, antioxidants and other nutrients. The old adage that we get everything from our diet and that supplementing with vitamins and minerals is just creating expensive urine has been knocked on the head. It is well researched that we no longer get everything we need nutritionally from our diet.

People who say that they are well off and eat a good diet, therefore they don't need supplements, don't always understand why they need antioxidants. Antioxidants scavenge free radicals a major source of which is the highly processed food of an affluent society.

Finally, if you do a vigorous exercise regime or play sports where a lot of activity is involved, then your body will generate further free radicals. In order to protect your cells, joints and tissues, it is advisable to increase your intake of antioxidants to counteract this extra free radical activity.

Understanding Free Radicals and Antioxidants

What are free radicals? Why do they damage the human body? How is it that vitamin A, E and C as well as beta carotene help protect the body from free radical damage? It is important to understand why eating at least five serving each day of antioxidant rich fruits and vegetables along with suitable antioxidant supplements will benefit your health, and help prevent cancer, heart disease and other illnesses from developing.

To start, let us look at free radicals. Where do they come from, and what damage do they do. Everyone has free radicals—they are part of living. They come from the metabolism of the food you eat as well as from environmental factors such as air pollution, radiation, cigarette smoke, herbicides, household cleaners, skin care products, cosmetics—in fact anything that has a chemical element in it. Even the immune system can develop free radicals to help destroy bacteria and viruses.

Free radicals are atoms or groups of atoms with an odd or un-paired number of electrons. These can be formed when oxygen interacts with certain molecules.

These highly reactive molecules can start a chain reaction—like a falling pack of cards. The danger is the damage they can do when they come into contact with important cellular components such as DNA or cell membranes. Cells can die if this occurs.

Some of the degenerative conditions caused by free radicals include:

- Deterioration of the eye lens, which contributes to cataracts or blindness.
- Inflammation of the joints (arthritis).
- Damage to nerve cells in the brain, which can result in Parkinson's or Alzheimer's disease.
- Acceleration of the aging process.
- Increased risk of coronary heart disease since free radicals encourage low-density lipoprotein (LDL) cholesterol to adhere to artery walls in the form of arterial plaque.
- Certain cancers triggered by damaged cell DNA.

This is where antioxidants come in. The main antioxidant vitamins are vitamin A, beta carotene, vitamin C and vitamin E. There are also antioxidant minerals such as selenium and zinc, and antioxidant herbs such as ginkgo biloba and garlic which support the circulatory system.

Antioxidants neutralize free radicals by donating one of their own electrons thus ending the electron stealing cycle. The antioxidants don't become free radicals themselves as they have spare electrons and are stable in either form. They act as protectors and help to prevent tissue and cell damage which could lead to various diseases.

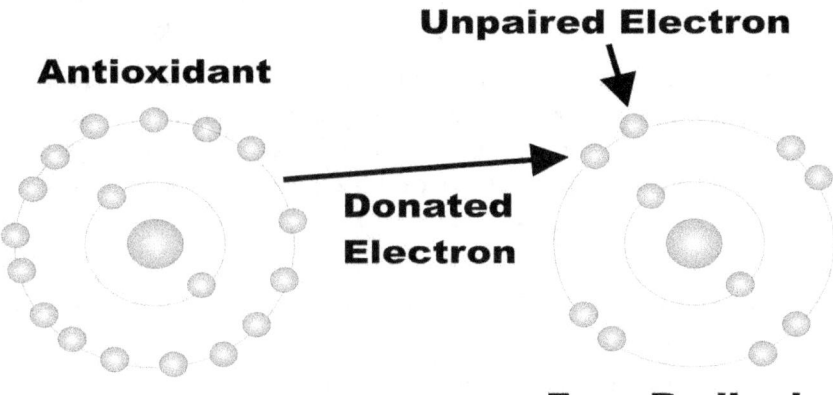

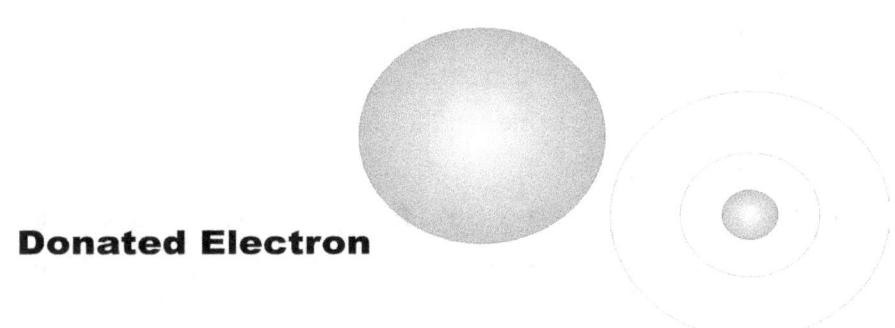

Antioxidants and Disease Prevention

The greatest killers in the Western world are heart disease, stroke and cancer. Vitamin E is the most abundant fat soluble antioxidant in the body. It is one of the main defenders against oxidation and helps protect you against cardiovascular disease by helping to neutralize the effects of LDL (low density lipoprotein)—the "bad" cholesterol and plaque formation which blocks arteries and can lead to a heart attack or stroke.

The most abundant water soluble antioxidant is vitamin C. Vitamin C helps to neutralize free radical formations caused by cigarette smoke and other forms of air pollution. Also many studies have shown that high doses of vitamin C equate to lower rates of cancer especially of the mouth, larynx and esophagus.

So, along with your five servings each day of antioxidant rich fruit and vegetables, you may want to consider topping up with extra antioxidant supplements: vitamin E, C and beta carotene as well.

Some good sources of antioxidants include:

- **Allium sulfur compounds**—leeks, onions and garlic
- **Anthocyanins**—eggplant, grapes and berries
- **Beta-carotene**—pumpkin, mangoes, apricots, carrots, spinach and parsley
- **Catechins**—red wine and green tea
- **Copper**—seafood, lean meat, milk and nuts
- **Cryptoxanthins**—red capsicum, pumpkin and mangoes
- **Flavonoids**—tea, green tea, citrus fruits, red wine, onion and apples
- **Indoles**—cruciferous vegetables such as broccoli, cabbage and cauliflower
- **Isoflavonoids**—soybeans, tofu, lentils, peas and milk
- **Lignans**—sesame seeds, bran, whole grains and vegetables
- **Lutein**—leafy greens like spinach and corn
- **Lycopene**—tomatoes, pink grapefruit and watermelon
- **Manganese**—seafood, lean meat, milk and nuts
- **Polyphenols**—thyme and oregano
- **Selenium**—seafood, offal, lean meat and whole grains
- **Vitamin C**—oranges, blackcurrants, kiwi fruit, mangoes, broccoli,

spinach, capsicum and strawberries

- **Vitamin E**—vegetable oils (such as wheat germ oil), avocados, nuts, seeds and whole grains

- **Zinc**—seafood, lean meat, milk and nuts

- **Zoochemicals**—red meat, offal, and fish. (Also derived from the plants that animals eat.)

The Need for Supplements

So let us now have a look at supplements and see where they fit in. The subject is so diverse as well as interesting.

One thing to understand is that all supplements are not created equal. There is a vast range available from health food stores, supermarkets, pharmacies and on the Internet. The base material differs also. Some are manufactured from chemical by-products (synthetic) while others are manufactured from natural ingredients.

You have to ask yourself this question. Do you think that something that is manufactured from chemical by-products in a laboratory will have as beneficial an effect in the body as something that is derived from a natural vegetable (or animal) source?

Various tests have been done on synthetic vitamin products and others have been done on natural ones. The natural ones have an "energy factor" which is not available in synthetic ones. Basically natural supplements are a living thing, while something that is synthetic is not.

Even amongst the natural ones, there are differences. It is all to do with the base material. Is it organic or wild crafted (obtained from the wild), or is it from sources that have been treated with chemical fertilizers and pesticides.

It has long been established that you do not get all your daily requirements of vitamins and minerals from the food you eat. This is due to the way crops are grown, the way they are processed and finally how the food that is derived from those crops is prepared in the home. In addition to that, intensive faming methods over the years have depleted the minerals in the soil to such an extent that hardly any exist anymore.

The following table give an example of how much mineral loss takes place in food processing and flour refining.

Percentage of Minerals Lost Through Food Processing			
	White Flour	Sugar Refining	Rice Polishing
Chromium	98%	78%	86%
Manganese	92%	54%	75%
Zinc	95%	88%	89%

Percentage of Minerals Lost Through Refining Flour			
Calcium	60%	Molybdenum	48%
Chromium	98%	Phosphorus	71%
Cobalt	89%	Potassium	77%
Copper	68%	Selenium	16%
Iron	76%	Sodium	78%
Magnesium	85%	Zinc	78%
Manganese	86%		

Interestingly, many of the vitamins that are so vital to your good health were only discovered less than 100 years ago. In fact most of the B vitamins were only identified in the 1920s and 1930s. Although not a vitamin, I have included Co-Q10 (Co-Enzyme Q10) which was only discovered in 1957 and is found in every cell of the human body. It is intimately linked to good heart health.

As research progresses, many more vitamins and minerals will be discovered and "named" as the years go by. The following table shows the relevant dates.

	Year Discovered		Year Discovered
Vitamin A	1912 - 1914	Vitamin B9	1933
Vitamin B1	1912	Vitamin B12	1948
Vitamin B2	1926	Vitamin C	1747 & 1912
Vitamin B3	1937	Vitamin D	1932
Vitamin B5	1933	Vitamin E	1922
Vitamin B6	1934	Co-Q10	1957
Vitamin B7	1927		

A Basic Supplement

Selecting a supplement is difficult when you don't have a guide. After all, everyone who sells them says theirs is the best. That's why I worked out the following table to explain what a basic supplement should contain. The best supplement will have all the recognized vitamins and all the minerals except calcium and magnesium at 50 percent of the RDA. It will have some calcium and magnesium, but not 50 percent of the RDA; possibly only 15 percent. The reason is simple: you need so much of these two minerals that they simply won't fit in a pill that contains everything else.

Take a look at the table on the next page. The middle column shows the amount of the nutrient you should get in a supplement. The end columns show it as a percentage of the UK and the USA RDA for average adults.

If you search the pharmacy and health food stores for exactly the same supplement shown in this table, you probably won't find one. Don't despair; simply come as close as possible to it. You might find all the vitamins and minerals, except calcium and magnesium. Take calcium and magnesium as a separate supplement.

The supplement should contain the nutrients shown in the table, in approximately the same ratios to one another; that is the most important criteria—that it is balanced.

Selecting a calcium and mineral supplement depends on the number of dairy products you use and how much your basic supplement contains. If you don't take milk, yogurt or cheese make up for it with a supplement that supplies at least 600mg of calcium and 200mg of magnesium daily. These two essential minerals should not be overlooked.

Is more better? More of some nutrients can help. Compare your body maintenance with that of your car. Keep your car well tuned and serviced and it will respond well to good fuel. Neglect it and you may as well use the cheapest fuel available. If you follow the use of the sensible supplements outlined, you will do just fine. If you feel better using more of some nutrients, it is okay; after all, you are a unique individual and have your own needs.

To sum it all up, natural foods are balanced in fat, protein and carbohydrates and the minerals potassium and sodium. If you eat a wide variety, you will get all your vitamins, minerals and fiber along with your supplement regime. It is important too, that you know what foods cause stress on your body due to a vitamin/mineral imbalance, so that you can avoid them.

An Excellent Supplement			
Nutrient: Vitamins/ Minerals	Supplement Amount	% of UK RDA	% of USA RDA
Vitamin A *RE	500mcg	63	56
Vitamin D	5mcg	100	33
Vitamin E	5mg	42	33
Vitamin C	30mg	38	33
Vitamin B1	0.8mg	73	66
Vitamin B2	0.8mg	57	62
Vitamin B3	10mg	63	62
Vitamin B6	1.4mg	100	108
Vitamin 9	150mcg	75	38
Vitamin B12	1.0mcg	40	42
Calcium	400mg	50	40
Magnesium	200mg	50	50
Iron	6mg	43	75
Zinc	8mg	80	73
Iodine	75mcg	50	50
*RE = Retinol Equivalent			

Enzymes

We also need enzymes—all living things contain enzymes. Enzymes work as catalysts and produce energy. Enzymes are capable of performing these tasks because, unlike food proteins such as caseine in egg albumin, gelatin, or soy protein, they are catalysts. This means that by their mere presence, and without being consumed in the process, enzymes can speed up chemical processes that would otherwise run very slowly, if at all. So in a nutshell, unlike vitamins and minerals, which are the building blocks of various body functions, enzymes are the body's workers—they make things happen. But very few people know about the vital role that enzymes play in maintaining a healthy body.

There are three broad classifications of enzymes: those that are contained naturally in the food itself, those that are manufactured by the body and assist in the breakdown and assimilation of food, and metabolic enzymes that provide chemical interactions within the body.

Each enzyme is designed to do a specific job. A protease enzyme (which breaks down protein) will not break down carbohydrates; likewise an enzyme whose job it is to break down milk sugar and milk protein (a job for lactase) will not break down fats (that is a job for lipase).

Nature planned for food enzymes to play an important role in the digestion of our food. Scientists say that digestive problems are a major health hazard in modern society. To explain the importance of enzymes is not easy, but my goal is to present an understanding of the role that enzymes play in keeping you healthy.

All raw, uncooked fruit, vegetables, meat, and poultry contain enzymes that will digest the food in which they are contained. The problem is that processing these foods destroys most of the enzymes. If food enzymes do some of the work, the body is not burdened with eliminating an accumulation of food it cannot assimilate.

Food allergies, gas and bloating, heartburn, and constipation or diarrhea are problems that can result from a lack of enzymes. Studies are gradually revealing that the resulting metabolic problems may be the direct cause of many chronic degenerative diseases.

To ensure that you get adequate enzymes, it is preferable to take enzyme supplements. These usually come in either enteric coated capsules (enteric meaning it will dissolve in the stomach or small intestine, and not before it gets to where it is supposed to work) or in tablet form.

Full spectrum enzyme supplements are available which means they contain enzymes that will assist in the breakdown of protein, carbohydrates, fats and starches. You may also see "proteolytic enzymes". These are in fact protease enzymes that break down proteins into their smallest elements. There are a large selection of enzyme supplements available, make sure you purchase one that is manufactured by a reputable supplier.

Sometimes an enzyme formula will contain hydrochloric acid (a stomach acid), which helps in the breakdown of foods in the stomach. As a person gets older, the body produces less of this acid, which can result in digestive problems and malabsorption of nutrients. If you have eaten a meal and feel as if you have a heavy weight in your stomach, then you may be lacking hydrochloric acid.

Here is a list of the main digestive enzymes and their function:

- **Alpha galactosidase** aids in the breakdown of complex carbohydrates commonly found in fruits and vegetables.
- **Amylase** (Mycozyme) digests starches.
- **Bile Salts** emulsify fats and prepare them for further digestion by the enzyme Lipase.
- **Cellulase** helps breakdown the cellular structure of plant fibers.
- **Glucoamylase** digests glucose sugars.
- **Invertase** aids in the breakdown of table sugar (sucrose).
- **Lactase** aids in the breakdown of milk sugar and milk protein.
- **Lipase** assists in the breakdown of dietary fats.
- **Malt Diastase** aids in the support of digestion and general nutrition.
- **Pancreatin** is produced by the pancreas to digest proteins, carbohydrates, and fats in the small intestine.
- **Papain** and **Bromelain** digest proteins.
- **Pepsin** is used for the digestion of proteins.
- **Peptidase** aids in the breakdown of proteins.
- **Protease** aids in the breakdown of proteins.

Amino Acids – The Building Blocks of Proteins

Amino Acids are the building blocks (and play a central role) in the make-up of proteins. They also have a secondary role to play in metabolism.

Various proteins make up muscles, tendons, organs, glands, hair, and nails. Proteins not only act as catalysts in the reactions of living cells, but they are also responsible for growth, maintenance and repair of cells too.

Amino acids form antibodies to combat bacteria and viruses that invade the body, and they form part of the enzyme and hormonal system too. Additional activities of amino acids include: building nucleoproteins (RNA and DNA), and carrying oxygen around the body.

Water makes up the largest portion of human body-weight; the next largest portion is made up of proteins.

There are two types of amino acids: essential amino acids which must be obtained from the diet as the body cannot manufacture them itself, and non-essential amino acids which the body can manufacture.

Of the 21 amino acids, 9 of these are essential amino acids. If one of the essential amino acids is missing in the diet, then degradation of body protein's will occur in such areas as muscles, tendons or nails etc..

Essential amino acids are not stored in the body for use later, (unlike fat and starch) and must be included in the diet each day.

Food sources of amino acids include: meat, poultry, fish, eggs, dairy products, grains, legumes, beans, and nuts. However, if they are lacking in the diet, then the essential ones can be taken as a supplement by capsule or tablet.

The following is a list of amino acids and their function in the human body.

Essential Amino Acids:

Histidine

Histidine is sometimes classed as an essential amino acid. It is found as part of hemoglobin; it has been used for the treatment of rheumatoid arthritis, allergies, ulcers and anemia. It is used for the treatment of digestive ulcers; it is also responsible for the manufacture of red and white blood cells. This amino acid is important for growth and repair of tissues; and is essential for the maintenance of the myelin sheaths which protects nerve cells.

It is a major protector of the body from radiation damage. It assists in lowering blood pressure, and helps in the removal of heavy metals from the body. In addition it facilitates in sexual arousal.

Isoleucine

Helps in the formation of hemoglobin. It is a regulator of blood sugar and a facilitator of energy in the muscle tissues, in addition to being a repair agent for bone, muscle tissue and skin. Isoleucine is often deficient in debilitated individuals.

Leucine

Works with Isoleucine and Valine to promote the healing of muscle tissue breakdown, skin, and broken bones. It acts as a moderator for the uptake of neurotransmitter precursors by the brain to slow the passage of pain signals to the nervous system.

Leucine is recommended for individuals in post-surgery recovery, and for helping to lower blood sugar levels. It acts as an assistant for increasing the production of growth hormones.

Lysine

Ensures an adequate absorption of calcium. It assists in the formation of collagen which forms bones, cartilage and connective tissues. In addition, it helps with the formation of antibodies, hormones and enzymes, which are active fighters against herpes, viral growth and cold sores. It also helps to lower high serum triglyceride levels.

When Lysine is combined with vitamin C, it forms L. Carnitine—a biochemical agent that enables tissue in the muscles to use oxygen more efficiently thus warding off the effects of chronic fatigue.

Methionine

A strong antioxidant and an excellent way to obtain sulfur, that helps prevent problems of the hair, skin pores, and also fingernails. It aids with the breakdown of fats, therefore helping avoid a build-up of fat within the liver and arteries which may prevent the flow of blood to the brain, heart, and kidneys.

Methionine helps to detox harmful agents such as lead along with other heavy metals. It aids in reducing muscle weakness; and helps prevent brittle hair; as well as providing a safeguard against the effects often associated with radiation.

It assists women who take oral birth control pills as it encourages the excretion of estrogen. In addition, it reduces the level of histamine in the body that may cause the brain to relay incorrect communications. Furthermore it is also helpful to individuals experiencing schizophrenia. Methionine is a precursor of cysteine (a sulfur non-essential amino acid) and creatine. It increases levels of glutathione (a powerful antioxidant) and reduces blood cholesterol levels.

Phenylalanine

Manufactures norepinephrine—a neurotransmitter (chemical) that passes messages between nerve cells in the brain. One of its functions is to enhance alertness and wakefulness, as well as boosting memory and reducing pain. Furthermore, it curbs hunger pains and forms a major part of collagen production, in addition to suppressing appetite. It is used to treat arthritis and depression as well as certain motor neuron diseases.

Threonine

Helps in the maintenance of a proper protein balance in the body, in addition to being involved in the formation of collagen, elastin and tooth enamel. It assists in the assimilation of nutrients from food and in metabolism. When it is combined with methionine and aspartic acid (a non-essential amino acid), it blocks the build-up of fats in the liver.

Tryptophan

Tryptophan is especially useful to control hyperactivity in children. As it is a natural relaxant, it helps reduce insomnia by encouraging normal sleep patterns. Tryptophan also eases the effects of anxiety and depression and enhances mood. It acts as an appetite suppressant and is therefore useful in a weight control, program. In addition, it aids in the proper functioning of the immune system and improves the release of growth hormones.

Valine

Valine does a lot of work especially with regard to muscles where it is involved in metabolism, coordination and supplying energy to muscle tissue. It is involved in maintaining a proper nitrogen balance in the body as well as being a treatment for liver and gallbladder disease. It also works in the nervous system where it calms emotions and encourages vigor.

Non-Essential Amino Acids:

Alanine

This non-essential amino acid is needed if a person does aerobic exercise as it guards against a toxic build-up in muscle cells which is generated when exercising and more energy is expended by the body. Alanine also plays a role in glucose metabolism that the body converts to energy.

Arginine

Often used in an erectile dysfunction program, arginine increases blood flow to the penis, in addition to increasing sperm count; it is very important for proper functioning of the immune system, especially in retardation of tumor growth and cancer proliferation. It stimulates the thymus gland to make T cells—a vital constituent of the immune system. In addition, it promotes the release of insulin from the pancreas, as well as reducing alcohol toxicity and neutralizing ammonia.

In a weight loss program it is important for reducing body fat and increasing muscle mass. It assists in the discharge of growth hormones to facilitate muscle growth and tissue repair.

Arginine is an important constituent of collagen which makes it especially useful for arthritic conditions and inflamed tissue disorders.

Aspartic Acid

Is involved in the function of RNA and DNA which are transporters of genetic information such as identity. It also acts as a carrier of specific minerals through the small intestine into the bloodstream for use by body cells. Aspartic Acid is intimately involved in revitalizing cell formation and activity, as well as being involved in metabolism.

It merges with other amino acids to create molecules that absorb and remove toxins from the bloodstream. In addition, it also purges ammonia from the liver.

As it is also involved in increasing stamina, it is excellent for those suffering from chronic fatigue and depression.

Cysteine

I have always had an interest in the actions of sulfur compounds in the body, and here we have cysteine (or to give it its full name, N-acetyl cysteine (NAC)—a sulfur non-essential amino acid—that is linked to the essential (sulfur) amino acid methionine. Another sulfur amino acid homocysteine is also involved here too.

Homocysteine is a harmful amino acid which is not obtained from the diet. Instead, it is synthesized from methionine by the addition of adenosine triphosphate (ATP). ATP is responsible for transporting chemical energy within cells for metabolism. The addition of ATP creates a catalytic action to form S-adenosylmethionine (SAMe). This is an intermediate process which ultimately forms homocysteine.

Homocysteine has two main roles: It can be converted back to methionine with the aid of vitamin B12 (cyanocobalamin) or used to create cysteine and alpha-ketobuterate with the aid of vitamin B6 (pyridoxine) and vitamin B9 (folic acid).

If B vitamins are lacking in the body, then the conversion of homocysteine back to methionine or to cysteine can be greatly reduced. If this happens, then homocysteine will form a sticky plaque on arterial walls. For this reason, it is linked to an increased risk of heart disease, stroke and dementia. Additionally homocysteine levels rise with age and if a person smokes.

Cysteine has important functions to perform, including: acting as a powerful antioxidant and protector of the liver and brain from the effects of alcohol, drugs and smoking.

Cysteine also helps prevent hardening of the arteries and eases the pain of rheumatoid arthritis. Additionally, it helps burn fat and builds muscle, as well as facilitating recovery from burns.

Glutamic Acid

Glutamic Acid acts as a fuel for the brain by increasing mental capacity in addition to being an excitatory neurotransmitter for the nervous system and spinal cord. It is important for sugar and fat metabolism, and is a carrier of potassium into the spinal fluid. It helps correct personality disorders and is a precursor of arginine, glutamine, glutathione, ornothine, proline, and gamma-amino-butyric acid (GABA)—a neurotransmitter that is synthesized in the brain.

Glutamine

The most abundant amino acid which plays a critical role in immune system performance. It is used along with Omega-3 essential fatty acids to treat a leaky gut. It has an important role to play in building and maintaining muscle tissue. Additionally, it helps prevent muscle wasting that can be the result of extended bed rest or such diseases as AIDS and cancer.

Glutamine is important for maintaining the pH (acid/alkaline balance) of the body as well as assisting in maintaining digestive and intestinal system health.

It is also considered a "brain food" as it assists in memory function and concentration, as well as providing a source of energy. In addition, it relieves instances of impotence and fatigue.

Glycine

Especially useful to calm aggressive and manic depressive individuals.

It is involved in supporting a healthy nervous system and assists in making several other amino acids. It is an integral part of hemoglobin and cytochromes—enzymes which are involved in energy production. Glycine is involved in the manufacture of glucagon which activates glycogen for energy.

Ornithine

Assists in stimulating the release of growth hormones which encourages the metabolism of body fat. This effect is increased with the addition of arginine and carnitine.

Ornithine is an important component of a strong immune system as well as being involved in purging ammonia, and liver regeneration.

It facilitates insulin secretion and assists insulin's vocation as a muscle building hormone.

Proline

Partners with vitamin C to elevate healthy connective tissue. It enhances skin texture by assisting with the production of collagen to replace collagen that is lost through aging. Proline plays a role in cartilage healing and reinforcement of joints, tendons and the heart muscle.

Serine

Serine is a part of the myelin sheaths that cover and protect nerve fibers. It is a component in DNA and RNA function (which are transporters of genetic information such as identity), as well as cell formation.

It supports the immune system by producing immunoglobulins and antibodies to fight infections. In addition, it helps metabolize fats and fatty acids as well as being a storage source of glucose by the liver and muscles.

Taurine

Taurine is critical for the proper utilization of calcium, magnesium, potassium and sodium. It is a key component of good vision by helping prevent macular degeneration. It is also an important component of bile which is required by the digestive system to break down fats.

Taurine aids in the cleansing of free radical waste and helps control many aspects of the aging process within the body. It is important for circulatory system health for those people who suffer from atherosclerosis, cardiac arrhythmias or hypertension (high blood pressure).

Taurine provides neurotransmitter activity in areas of the brain and retina.

Tyrosine

Tyrosine is important for the correct functioning of the glandular and nervous systems. As a regulator of mood and depressive tendencies, tyrosine is a precursor of adrenaline, norepinephrine and dopamine, and works with the thyroid, adrenal and pituitary glands to fulfill this role.

It contains melanin which is the pigment responsible for hair and skin color.

It also assists in cases of chronic fatigue and low sex drive, allergies and headaches.

Herbs—An Ancient, Natural Medicinal Treatment

Herbal medicine is the oldest known form of healthcare. Whether it is Western natural medicine, or Chinese, Indian or Native American, herbal combinations are used to improve the performance of various organs.

The Chinese emperor Shen Nong (who lived around 5000BC) wrote a treatise on herbs that is still in use today. For example, Shen Nong recommended the use of Ma Huang (known as ephedra in the Western world), to treat respiratory problems. Ephedrine, extracted from ephedra, has been widely used as a decongestant.

In another example, King Hammurabi of Babylon (c.1800B.C.) recommended the use of mint for digestive disorders. Today, peppermint is widely used to relieve nausea – especially travel sickness and vomiting.

The Middle East in particular has a rich history of herbal healing. Surviving texts from the ancient people's of Mesopotamia, Egypt, and India explain with words and pictures how to use medicinal plant products, such as castor oil, linseed oil, and white poppies.

During the Middle Ages, most households would have an extensive herb garden which was used to treat all the family's ailments. Home grown herbal plants were the only form of medicine available. The medicinal uses for these herbal plants were passed from generation to generation within a family by word of mouth.

In Europe, in 1649, Nicholas Culpeper wrote A Physical Directory and a few years later The English Physician. This herbal pharmacopeia was one of the first manuals that anyone could use for health care, and it is still often quoted from today.

In the nineteenth century, Western medicine as we know it today, progressed from being passed on from generation to generation where everyone who was interested had medicinal knowledge, to the realm of just a few that had a more scientific background.

This came about by scientific methods being developed to extract and synthesize active ingredients in plants to manufacture drugs. And a huge and powerful drugs industry was born.

Herbal plants contain many different compounds: active ingredients in the form of alkaloids, volatile oils, vitamins, minerals, glycosides, bioflavonoids, and other ingredients that are important in supporting a particular herbs medicinal qualities. Some of these substances have been identified, but many more have yet to be discovered.

The problem that then arises is when drugs are manufactured; an active ingredient is extracted and synthesized in a laboratory to emulate the natural herb. But all the other ingredients in the plant are left behind. These "other ingredients" play the role of a natural safeguard which is lost.

By comparison, it usually takes a larger amount of a whole herb, with all of its components, to reach a toxic level. The end result with the drug and its isolated active ingredient is that some of these substances can become toxic in small amounts, which can cause serious side effects from the use of these drugs.

Interestingly, watching drug commercials on TV here in the United States, most of the time is taken up with all the side effects which the drug can cause.

Today components from plants form the basis of many medications used for such conditions as asthma, high blood pressure and heart disease to name a few.

Two examples: salicylic acid, a precursor of aspirin, was originally derived from white willow bark and the meadowsweet plant. Digitalis which is derived from the foxglove plant has been used for many years as a heart medication.

Herbs generally fall into two categories those that grow in the wild and are called wild crafted. These are harvested where the plant grows in its natural habitat. The other is commercially grown, where a greater control over quality and growing conditions can be exercised.

Herbal products are available in several forms: liquid, tablets, capsules, extracts, tinctures, teas, salves, ointments, fresh, or as dried plant parts. Some are supplied as single herbs while others are made into combinations to treat a specific condition.

Capsules and Tablets

The herb is ground into a very fine powder and then either inserted into a capsule or pressed into a tablet form. Generally, herbs in capsules and tablets are less potent than tinctures or extracts. Additionally, read the label to make sure no fillers have been added. Fillers could be either natural or synthetic.

Extracts

Extracts can be used internally and externally. Externally, they can be rubbed into the skin to treat arthritic conditions or strained muscles and ligaments. Internally, they can be used for a variety of health conditions.

Extracts can be made with alcohol, like tinctures, or glycerin or water can be used. The herb is in a concentrated form and is easily assimilated. The only way to tell what method has been used is to read the label.

Lozenges

Lozenges are often sucked to ward off the effects of a cold or cough, or they may be used as a decongestant. Many are fortified with vitamin C. Read the label to make sure they are not coated with refined sugar or an artificial sweetener.

Ointments, Salves, and Rubs

There are many products available in your health food store to treat burns, wounds, skin rashes and insect bites, or as heat producing herbs to treat sprains, pulled muscles or to relax muscle aches.

Teas

A huge selection of herbal teas is available either from your health food store or supermarket. Herbal teas take several forms from being relaxing, comforting or having medicinal properties. They come either as loose tea or in tea bags. Either way, they just need preparing with hot water for a very beneficial drink.

Tinctures

A tincture usually contains alcohol which is used to extract and concentrate the active properties of the herb. Tinctures are very easily assimilated by the body and are therefore a very easy and effective way to take a herbal product. If you wish to lessen the effect of the alcohol, then pour the tincture into a small amount of very hot water for a few minutes. The alcohol will vaporize and after it has cooled, it will be ready to drink.

Herbal products, unlike drugs, will take time to provide a beneficial effect in the body. The time scale could be a few weeks to a few months, depending on what the herbal preparation is being used for.

The reason for this is that the herb will supply various "actions" in the body. First a cleansing or neutralizing action. Next possibly an antiseptic action, followed by a deodorizing action, and finally a building action to re-build the body back to full health. As you can appreciate, all this takes time, but it is well worth the wait in the long run.

The quality of the raw material used will determine the potency of the finished herbal product. Therefore it is well worth while doing a little research on a particular supplier or manufacturer before you part with your money.

An A to Z of Herbs

Alfalfa

Alfalfa is a grass which contains all the essential amino acids as well as being rich in trace minerals and enzymes. It is frequently taken to lessen the effects of hay fever allergies. It is also fed to horses as a counter to arthritic conditions and digestive problems.

As it is a good source of fiber, it is useful for detoxifying the body in addition to improving liver health.

Black Cohosh

Black Cohosh is widely used to treat menopausal symptoms such as hot flashes, night sweats, migraines, mood swings, heart palpitations and dryness. The roots of the plant are used medically and are available as capsules, a liquid extract or tablets.

Black Walnut

Traditionally used as a nutritional aid for the intestinal system, Black Walnut has the same laxative action as Cascara Sagrada, but it works more gently. Due to its astringent qualities, Black Walnut has the power to assist the body in protecting itself from harmful agents such as parasitic worms. It also has a high iodine content, which is good for energy as it supports thyroid function.

Buchu

Buchu is native to South Africa, where it was used by native people as well as early colonists as a treatment for urinary tract infections. It has also been used for arthritis, cholera, kidney stones and muscle aches. Buchu is often combined with Cranberry where it acts as a diuretic and improves digestion. Buchu works best in acidic urine conditions.

Burdock Root

Burdock Root is one of the best blood purifiers to clear circulatory and lymphatic congestion. As it assists in alleviating excess body fluids, toxins are more easily purged from the body.

Other uses for Burdock Root: aids in reducing swelling around joints, expels surplus calcium deposits and cleanses the blood of harmful acids.

Capsicum

Capsicum also called cayenne has a warming effect and is often used to treat instances of cold hands and cold feet. As such it is an excellent circulatory product. It has also gained a good reputation as a painkiller and digestive aid. The main active ingredient is capsaicin—an oily phytochemical. Additionally, it has been used to relieve symptoms of a cold and sore throat.

Cascara Sagrada

Well known for it quick acting laxative effects. It is often used for constipation in addition to helping purge toxins from the body. It promotes peristaltic action—the movement of waste matter through the colon, and stimulates secretions from the gall bladder, liver, pancreas and stomach.

Chamomile

Dried Chamomile flowers were used in ancient Egypt, Greece and Rome to treat many disorders of the body including anxiety, stress and sleeping problems. This was achieved by its calming and sedative effect. In more recent times it has been used as a tea for relaxation and as a sleep aid.

Chickweed

Chickweed is used to strengthen the colon and stomach as well as helping to dissolve plaque and fatty deposits. Chickweed has healing properties for stomach ulcers and inflammation in the colon.

Cloves

Cloves are a good natural parasite cleansing herb which can be obtained as a liquid, powder or in a capsule.

Cranberry

Cranberry's main purpose is to treat bacterial infections in the bladder. It is often combined with Buchu herb.

When used together, these two herbs have anti-inflammatory, diuretic and antiseptic properties. Scientific studies show that Cranberry makes the urinary tract inhospitable to bacteria, lessening the risk of urinary tract infections. Buchu acts as a diuretic and improves digestion. This product works best in acidic urine conditions.

Dandelion

Dandelion has been used for centuries to stimulate the liver to detoxify poisons. It is important for promoting good circulatory system function and strengthening weak arteries.

Dong Quai

Dong Quai—a member of the celery family—is one of the oldest known herbs, having been used in China, Japan and Korea for over 1,000 years. It is primarily known as a women's product, to relieve menopausal symptoms such as: hot flashes, menstrual disorders such as cramps, irregular menstrual cycles, infrequent periods, premenstrual syndrome (PMS), and menopausal symptoms.

It is suggested that Dong Quai contains compounds that may help reduce pain, dilate blood vessels, and stimulate and relax uterine muscles.

In traditional Chinese medicine (TCM), different parts of the Dong Quai root are used for different actions in the body: the root head is used as an anticoagulant, the main part of the root is used as a tonic, and the tail-end of the root is used to remove blood stagnation. Because it is a balancer of the female hormonal system, it is often called "female's ginseng."

Echinacea

There are various strains of Echinacea. It is used to support the immune system and is involved in the production of white blood cells, which assists the body in fighting infection. Echinacea purges toxins from the blood and enhances lymphatic drainage.

Echinacea contains polysaccharides that stimulate the production of phagocytes (cells that engulf and consume foreign matter) and activate T-lymphocytes, macrophages and natural killer cells. Taken at the earliest sign of a cold or infection, Echinacea may help cut recovery time considerably.

Elderberry

One of the oldest known herbs. It works in the respiratory and immune body systems, and is usually used to counter the effects of colds, flu, congestion, sore throat and inflammation.

Fennel Seed

Fennel Seed has several uses including: supporting the digestive and nervous systems, alleviating the effects of colic, gas and intestinal problems. It also has diuretic properties.

Fenugreek

Fenugreek comprises various components including saponins, alkaloids and fiber. It is a respiratory system herb which assists in expelling mucous, phlegm and infections from the lungs, and toxic waste through the lymphatic system. In addition, Fenugreek is able to dissolve a hardened build up of mucous which can then be eliminated.

Garcinia Cambogia

Garcinia Cambogia is a tropical fruit which contains HCA (hydroxy-citric acid), which stimulates the body to burn carbohydrates as energy rather than storing them as fat. HCA acts as an appetite suppressant which reduces the intake of food, thus reducing fat and cholesterol formation.

Garlic

This popular herb offers a boost to the immune system with its antibacterial, antifungal and antiviral properties. It is excellent for purging candida yeast and parasites from the body.

Garlic has so many uses from using it in cooking to it being an excellent product for heart health. Other recognized health benefits of Garlic include, acting as an antibiotic and having anti-cholesterol and anti-hypertensive properties.

It is also an antioxidant which protects the body against the effects of free radical damage. Its high sulfur content assists in cell purification.

Allicin is the principle biologically active compound which gives Garlic its odor. Be warned, many so called "odorless" Garlic products have the active compound removed which makes it rather worthless. It can be obtained as a Garlic bulb, in a capsule or in tablet form.

Garlic has many uses:

- Antibiotic—natural penicillin
- Arteriosclerosis
- Arthritis
- Asthma
- Blood poisoning
- High blood pressure
- Anti-viral
- Anti-bacterial
- Destroys many types of parasites
- For respiratory conditions use with Mullein or Lobelia
- As a decongestant / expectorant use with Lobelia
- For bacterial infection use with Golden Seal, Echinacea, Pau d'Arco
- For viral infection use with Colloidal Silver

- For yeast infections use with Pau d'Arco
- For swollen lymph nodes use with Lobelia and Mullein
- For parasites use with Pumpkin Seeds and Black Walnut

Gentian Root

Gentian Root helps in the breakdown of fats and proteins and assists in the body's assimilation of iron and vitamin B12. As it has a cooling effect on body tissue, this helps reduce infections and inflammation. Gentian Root also promotes digestive secretions.

Ginger Root

Ginger Root is an excellent cleansing agent for the colon, skin and kidneys. It provides support to the respiratory system, and is often used to alleviate the effects of a cold or flu. Many people take it as a natural alternative for motion and morning sickness.

Ginkgo Biloba

Ginkgo Biloba—an antioxidant herb—promotes increased circulation. It also dilates blood vessels and bronchioles to improve circulation and oxygenation of cells. It also has scientifically proven nervous-system benefits in addition to improving memory function.

Golden Seal

Golden Seal has infection-fighting abilities and anti-inflammatory properties. It can be used as an alternative to Cranberry if required.

Grapefruit Seed Extract

Grapefruit Seed Extract is an effective anti-parasitic herb which has a very bitter taste. This can be sweetened by adding a small amount of honey.

Gymnema Sylvestre

Gymnema Sylvestre is a climbing plant which is native to Australia, parts of Africa and central and southern India, and is used in Ayurvedic medicine. It is primarily used for weight management to control appetite and cravings, but has also been used to treat constipation and diabetes

Hawthorn Berries

Hawthorn is known as the heart herb. It improves circulation and heart strength. In studies, hawthorn recipients also reported fewer overall symptoms, less fatigue and less shortness of breath.

It is often taken along with Ginkgo Biloba to improve circulation especially to the heart.

Hibiscus Flower

Hibiscus Flower has anti-bacterial properties as well as being an anti-parasitic. In addition it acts as a diuretic and has a soothing effect on the body.

Horsetail

This herb has diuretic properties and can help with some kidney conditions. It is particularly effective for healing when blood is present in the urine. Horsetail also has astringent properties and as such, is used for bed-wetting in children and incontinence in Adults.

Horsetail is rich in silica, which helps to soothe and strengthen connective tissue. Silica is required for bone and cartilage formation, as well as assisting the body in absorbing and utilizing calcium. Calcium is needed for repairing fractures and treating bone diseases, including rickets and osteoporosis. Horsetail is used to strengthen bones, teeth, nails and hair. The improved cartilage helps to lessen inflammation and combat joint pain, arthritis, gout, muscle cramps, hemorrhoids, spasms and rheumatism.

The silica content in Horsetail also promotes the growth of collagen, which is a protein found in connective tissue, Collagen assists in improving skin health and tone.

Kava Kava

Kava Kava is very effective at treating anxiety and depression. It has a natural sedative effect which does not affect alertness unlike some medications. It should not be taken for more than six months at a time unless advised otherwise by a qualified practitioner.

Korean Ginseng

Korean Ginseng—also called Panax Ginseng—has been used for over 5,000 years as a preventative tonic to nourish the whole body, especially for stress, fatigue and weak conditions. It grows primarily in China, South Korea and Japan.

Korean Ginseng is considered the strongest form of ginseng. Ginsenoside compounds assist in lowering blood sugar levels, while polysaccharides help to enhance the immune system. Korean Ginseng's antioxidant properties help to stimulate the immune system to help protect the body from various diseases and stress.

Korean Ginseng assists in the production of endorphins which makes a person feel exhilarated. It also has significant sexual health benefits to help improve erectile function, as well as increasing testosterone levels and sperm count.

Kudzu

Historically Asian-Healers have used Kudzu to treat colds, flu, high blood pressure, allergies and many other ailments.

More recently, Chinese-Healers have used Kudzu to treat people who have an alcohol dependency. It has also been used with St John's Wort to treat the depressive effects of alcohol withdrawal. Kudzu is available in capsules, tablets, and dried root.

Lavender

Lavender can be used in different ways to treat anxiety, tension, headaches and insomnia. It is usually steeped in hot water so that the steam can be inhaled. Other options are to make it into a tea or it can be used as an essential oil and massaged into the skin. This will help manage stress and improve mood, concentration and reduce anxiety. Lavender has the ability to relax the nervous system and improve sleep patterns.

Lemon Balm

Lemon Balm is a calmative for the nerves and as a result, relieves tension in the body. Its effect is soothing and is used for treating anxiety and stress.

Licorice Root

Licorice has long been recognized for the natural sweetness of its deep-sinking roots. Next to ginseng, licorice is the most popular herb used in Chinese formulas. It helps support the adrenal glands during periods of stress.

Lobelia

Lobelia has a lengthy history of use as an herbal remedy for respiratory conditions such as asthma, bronchitis, pneumonia, and cough. Traditionally, Native Americans smoked Lobelia as a treatment for asthma. Today, some herbalists use Lobelia to help clear mucus from the respiratory tract, including the throat, lungs, and bronchial tubes. Additionally, Lobelia is used as part of a comprehensive treatment plan for asthma.

Maca

Maca, also known as Peruvian Ginseng is used to increase stamina, energy and sexual function in both men and women. In one study, researchers found that Maca may help alleviate sexual dysfunction caused by the use of selective-serotonin re-uptake inhibitors (SSRIs) which are used in the treatment of depression.

Marshmallow

This mucilant soothes the kidneys when they are irritated or inflamed. Marshmallow contains volatile oils and tannins that are responsible for its diuretic actions. It is especially helpful in passing kidney stones.

Milk Thistle

This natural support to the liver contains a mixture of bioflavonoids, including silymarin. Milk Thistle strengthens the liver against auto-intoxication and stimulates protein synthesis in liver cells, which generates DNA and RNA.

Mullein

Mullein has both mucilant and astringent properties. Its powerful healing abilities make it useful for healing weak lung tissue and chronic respiratory congestion. It has a proven expectorant action that likely arises from saponin compounds in the plant. Scientific studies suggest that the mucilage in Mullein protects mucous membranes, thus preventing cell invasion by viral allergens.

Nopal

Nopal or Mexican Cactus as it is sometimes called is traditionally used by the Mexicans as a food especially in salads. The nutritional factors in Nopal act in the bowel to prevent fat and excessive sugars from entering the bloodstream. By helping the body maintain balanced blood sugar levels, Nopal aids the body in its battle against obesity. Additionally, it is used as an anti-inflammatory, as a laxative and as a hypoglycemic vehicle for diabetes and gastritis.

Oatstraw

Oatstraw is a good source of minerals for nourishing bones, hair, skin and nails. It helps calm the nervous system and can assist in depressive and conditions of exhaustion.

Olive Leaf Extract

Olive Leaf Extract supports normal blood pressure and cholesterol levels and strengthens the immune system against viral and bacterial attacks.

Oregano

Available in either enteric coated (meaning it will burst in the body where it is supposed to), or in liquid form, Oregano possesses anti-inflammatory antiviral and anti-fungal properties which makes it especially useful for eradicating candida yeast.

Papaya

Papaya contains proteolytic enzymes that aid in the digestion of proteins; I have included a list of enzymes and their function in the body under the enzymes section in this book.

Parsley

Parsley is probably one of the best known herbs as it is used in culinary dishes as well as for medicinal uses. It comes in a variety of different "leaf types", from feather like to curled to flat. The flat leafed variety is most often used for medicinal purposes.

It is used to treat urinary tract infections, indigestion, to relieve the effects of gas and as a digestive aid. Additionally, it is a natural body deodorizer and eradicates bad breath.

Passion Flower

A natural sedative, passionflower will help you sleep without leaving a groggy feeling the next morning. It is beneficial for calming the nervous system, and for stress conditions.

Passion Flower slows the breakdown of neurotransmitters which pass chemical messages between the body's cells, as well as working with certain enzymes. It also assists in calming an irritable bowel, as well as killing certain bacteria.

Pau D'Arco

Pau D'Arco is native to South America. It contains a chemical called lapachol, which may provide nutritional support to the immune system. It is commonly used against many conditions of unwanted growth, including fungus, yeast and tumors as well as fungal infections. Historically, it has also been used to remedy the side effects of some antibiotics.

Peppermint

Peppermint stimulates the production of digestive fluids. It also eradicates bad breath and helps settle an upset stomach. If purchased in liquid form, then only tiny drops should be applied to water, otherwise it will be too strong.

Pumpkin Seeds

One of the best tasting of all the anti-parasite herbal products. The seeds can be eaten as a snack. In fact they taste so good that you cannot eat enough of them. Pumpkin Seeds are very effective against tapeworms as well as other types of parasites. They also serve as a good source of essential fatty acids (EFAs) which are essential for good health.

Pygeum

Obtained from the bark of the African Cherry Tree, Pygeum Extract is used to prevent and relieve benign prostatic hyperplasia (BPH). It contains anti-inflammatory phytosterol compounds in addition to triterpenoid compounds which have an anti-swelling effect.

Red Raspberry

This herb is renowned for its nutritional support of the female reproductive system. Red Raspberry is known to nourish and strengthen the uterus. A common backyard fruit bush, Red Raspberry is an excellent herbal source of iron, manganese and niacin. It also contains quantities of vitamins C, A, D, E and B, as well as phosphorus and calcium.

Rosemary

Rosemary, a member of the mint family is an excellent tonic and improves circulation and supports the nervous system as well as enhancing the memory. It complements other members of the mint family in addition to Lavender and other herbs. It can be used in various forms. For example:

Rosemary Leaf Extract

Rosemary Leaf Extract as well as being excellent for the nervous system, it also supports the digestive system where problems arise due to emotional stress. In addition, it is also an excellent antibacterial and has astringent properties.

Rosemary Tea

Rosemary Tea has been drunk for centuries to ease the effects of headaches as well as improving circulation and neutralizing some of the effects of memory loss. It can help when working long hours or studying to help keep the mind focused on the task at hand. Like Rosemary Leaf Extract, it is also beneficial for the digestive system. Cold Rosemary Tea can be used as an antibacterial mouth wash.

Saw Palmetto

Saw Palmetto is mainly used to treat benign prostatic hyperplasia (BPH).

BPH is a male condition which includes frequent urination, difficulty in fulfilling the urge to urinate, dribbling after urination, a weak urinary stream, and finally, waking up several times at night to urinate.

Siberian Ginseng

Siberian Ginseng (eleuthero) contains compounds called ginsenosides which alleviate stress and boost mental and physical performance. It has been used for centuries in Russia and China as an adaptogen—meaning, it allows the body to relax during stressful periods. It also helps balance neurotransmitters such as serotonin and dopamine in the brain. In addition to helping balance blood sugar levels, it also enhances a sense of well-being.

Skullcap

Skullcap is a member of the mint family and is traditionally used as a nerve tonic as well as a sedative for relieving anxiety and insomnia. In addition it relieves nervous exhaustion and supports the nervous system.

Slippery Elm

Slippery Elm is very soothing to inflamed tissue—especially in the gastrointestinal tract—and as a result, is excellent for tissue healing. It is easily digested and has good laxative properties.

St. John's Wort

This popular herb has gained national attention for its ability to alleviate mild to moderate depression. It contains an active constituent, hypericin, which appears to prolong the activity of serotonin (a neurotransmitter) in the brain. St. John's Wort may also lengthen the performance of dopamine and nor-epinephrine, two brain chemicals that are linked to depression. In Europe, many doctors prescribe this herb instead of prescription antidepressant drugs.

Note! You can find further details on Stress and Depression by reading my eBook *"An Easy Way to Understand Stress and Depression"*, which is available from the Kindle Store, or there is a download printable version available at www.wisdomforlifemedia.com.

Una de Gato (Cats Claw)

The bark of a vine from South America. Una de Gato provides beneficial alkaloids to stimulate the immune system. It is also used for the following:

- As a cancer therapy to reduce the side effects of chemotherapy.
- As an anti-inflammatory for all types of arthritis.

- As a bowel and stomach protector and cleanser, and to treat ulcerative colitis as well as stomach ulcers.

- To treat a variety of bowel problems including, but not limited to: Crohn's disease, diverticulitis and irritable bowel syndrome (IBS).

- An excellent general body tonic to tone and protect all body systems.

It is usually taken in capsule form.

Uva Ursi

Uva Ursi is used to treat cystitis—inflammation of the urinary tract. Arbutin is the main component of Uva Ursi. Arbutin is absorbed in the stomach where it is converted into a substance with antimicrobial, astringent and antimicrobial properties.

Arbutin's main purpose is to soothe irritation and reduce inflammation during urination, as well as to fight infections in the urinary tract.

It is important for the urine to be alkaline for Uva Ursi to work properly. The acid / alkaline balance (pH) can be determined by using a litmus paper test strip. If the urine is too acidic then it can be brought to an alkaline state by the use of alkalizing agents such as calcium, magnesium supplements, chlorophyll in liquid form (chlorophyll is derived from alfalfa), and by eating alkalizing foods such as tomatoes, and the majority of fruits and vegetables. This is by no means a complete list. Note. While most citrus fruits are acidic, when they have been digested they are alkaline forming.

Acidic foods to avoid include: beef, pork, lamb, butter, peanut butter, and many more. There are some excellent acid / alkaline food lists available on the Internet. Just type "acid alkaline food lists" into your search engine.

Valerian

Valerian Root—a natural plant calcium—is often used as a pain killer. It has been used for centuries to treat anxiety and insomnia, and is best taken before bedtime.

Violet Leaf

Is a good source of vitamin C and beta carotene (which the body converts to vitamin A as needed). Violet Leaf has antifungal properties in addition to being a diuretic and laxative.

White Willow Bark

The use of White Willow Bark goes back to the time of Hippocrates. This Greek physician wrote about the medicinal benefits of White Willow Bark in the 5th century B.C.

However, it was in 1829 that scientists in Europe identified salicin as being the active ingredient, which is converted in the body to salicylic acid.

It was used as a popular remedy for the relief of pain in such conditions as inflammation, fever, joint pain and osteoarthritis.

Extracting salicin from herbs was a time consuming process, so in 1852, German scientists developed a synthetic form of salicylic acid. Unfortunately this had a tendency to cause stomach ulcers and bleeding.

Eventually the German company Bayer developed a synthetic version being less harsh which they called acetylsalicylic acid (ASA). This was then manufactured under the trade name aspirin. Today, low dose soluble aspirin is recommended by doctors to reduce a person's risk of a heart attack or stroke by 50 percent. However, aspirin still has the stigma of being associated with causing stomach bleeding and irritating the stomach lining.

Many people prefer White Willow Bark to aspirin because it does not irritate the stomach lining. Researchers have identified a possible reason for this in that salicin found naturally in White Willow Bark is only converted to the acid form after it is absorbed by the stomach.

Additionally, there are other active compounds in natural White Willow Bark which are not in the synthetic salicin. And these additional compounds make the natural salicin more effective than the synthetic form.

Witch Hazel

Witch Hazel has excellent anti-inflammatory and antiseptic properties. As it has a high flavonoid content, this helps to heal damaged blood vessels.

Yellow Dock

Assists with elimination and is one of the best blood builders in the herbal arsenal.

Yerba Mate

A herb from South America which is used to boost energy and stamina, but unlike caffeine containing plants, Yerba Mate does not cause the jitters or shakes. Historically it has also been used to treat asthma and various allergies.

It is usually made into a tea by pouring hot water on to the leaves, and then it is left for 10 minutes before straining.

Yohimbe

A native to the Congo, Cameroon, Nigeria, and Gabon, Yohimbe is used to prevent depression as it inhibits monoamine oxidase (MAO). Additionally it is used to treat erectile dysfunction either as a single herb, or in combination with other herbs.

Yucca Root

Yucca Root is high in fiber content and as such, is an excellent herb for digestive and intestinal problems. It can rid the body of undigested waste toxins which reside in the colon and cause foul smelling gasses.

Historically, Yucca Root has been used as an anti-inflammatory and laxative agent that purges toxins from joints which if left untreated, can cause inflammation that then leads to joint problems such as arthritis. Yucca is also effective at eliminating toxins from the blood, kidneys, liver and lymph.

When buying any herbal product, make sure there are no artificial fillers or artificial sugar coatings which would be used as a sweetener.

The Body Systems

Functions of the Circulatory System

Basic Function

The circulatory system is responsible for transporting nutrients to the cells and removing waste from the cells.

After the lungs have replaced the "blue" venal blood with red (by replacing carbon dioxide with oxygen), the heart pushes it throughout the body via arteries.

Arteries

Are living tubes with an outer layer of muscle. They allow for nutrient delivery to be adjusted according to the part of the body that needs it most. This causes a change in blood pressure in that area. Extreme nervous tension may cause a general vessel contraction that makes blood pressure soar, causing the heart to work harder.

Capillaries

Are the tiniest blood vessels. They carry blood to the areas of the body farthest from the heart.

Veins

Carry blood, now devoid of oxygen and full of carbon dioxide and other cell wastes, away for cleansing in the kidneys and re-oxygenation in the lungs. One complete cycle takes about 20 seconds. One-way valves in the leg veins help ease the heart's work.

The Lymphatic System

Is completely separate from the blood system. It is still part of the circulatory system because it re-circulates blood plasma trapped in tissue spaces. Lymph fluid not only helps to clear the tissue spaces but forms an important part of the immune system.

Common Problems Associated With The Circulatory System:

- Cholesterol/triglyceride buildup
- Hypertension (High blood pressure)
- Arterial plaque
- Stress
- Poor circulation
- Heart disease

Lifestyle Suggestions:

- Eat low to moderate amounts of fat daily.

- Avoid saturated fats.
- Eat lots of fruits, vegetables, onions and garlic.
- Perform aerobic exercise, especially walking.
- Manage weight.
- Avoid stress.

Interesting Facts:

- Cholesterol is made by the cells of all animals; humans manufacture most of their own in the liver. Cholesterol levels become dangerous when vessels are unprotected from oxidation by low levels of vitamin E and other antioxidants.
- A recent survey found that only 4 percent of women believe heart disease to be a top health risk, when in fact 34 percent die from this cause alone.
- According to the American Heart Association, 50 percent of middle-aged Americans have dangerously high levels of blood cholesterol.

Supplements for Circulatory System Health

For Cholesterol:

Chinese Red Yeast Rice

Chinese Red Yeast Rice has been used very effectively to lower cholesterol levels. This is due to it containing a family of monacolins (polyketides) with the ability to inhibit cholesterol synthesis and lower plasma cholesterol levels.

Garlic

Garlic is excellent for purging candida yeast and parasites from the body. Garlic has so many uses from using it in cooking to it being an excellent product for heart health. It also has antibacterial, anti-fungus and antiviral properties. Other recognized health benefits of Garlic include, acting as an antibiotic and having anti-cholesterol and anti-hypertensive properties.

It is also an antioxidant which protects the body against the effects of free radical damage. Its high sulfur content assists in cell purification.

Allicin is the principle biological active compound which gives Garlic its odor. Be warned. Many so called "odorless" Garlic products have the active compound removed which makes it rather worthless. It can be obtained as a Garlic bulb, in a capsule or in tablet form.

Lecithin

Lecithin is an important phospholipid which is needed and utilized by all body cells as well as the heart, liver and kidneys. As it is a fat itself, it adheres to cell and nerve linings, forming a slippery barrier to prevent cholesterol and other fats from sticking. This ensures that blood flows more freely.

For The Heart:

Co-QIO

Co-Q10 is essential for generating energy in every body cell and may help prevent heart disease and hypertension. Co-Q10 is also an antioxidant and is used in dental practices to help fight gum disease. Statins—cholesterol lowering drugs, destroy Co-Q10, so anyone taking these drugs should consider supplementing with Co-Q10.

Ginkgo Biloba

Ginkgo Biloba promotes increased circulation. It also dilates blood vessels and bronchioles to improve circulation and oxygenation of cells. It also has scientifically proven nervous-system benefits in addition to improving memory function.

Hawthorn Berries

Hawthorn Berries are known as the heart herb. It improves circulation and heart strength. In studies, hawthorn recipients also reported fewer overall symptoms, less fatigue and less shortness of breath.

Hawthorn Berries are often taken along with Ginkgo Biloba to improve circulation especially to the heart.

Magnesium

This essential mineral keeps the heart muscle from going into spasm.

For Vascular Problems:
(Varicose Veins, Hemorrhoids, Spider Veins)

Butchers Broom

Butchers Broom has been used for hundreds of years to provide support to the circulatory system where it is used to strengthens blood vessel walls, making it ideal in cases of post-operative surgery to prevent thrombosis. It is also used to treat hemorrhoids, phlebitis and varicose veins.

Proanthocyanidins

Often sold under the trade name Pycnogenol. Proanthocyanidins are powerful antioxidants obtained from grape seed and pine bark. They help prevent cell damage by quenching oxidative free radicals. This combination of antioxidant nutrients has been shown to be many times more powerful than vitamin C or E. Proanthocyanidins also improve the integrity of collagen fibers, strengthening tissues in the skin, blood vessels, muscles, cartilage and other connective tissues.

Problems with Circulation:
(High Blood Pressure, Cold Hands and Feet, Hardening of the Arteries)

Capsicum

Capsicum also called cayenne has a warming effect and is often used to treat instances of cold hands and cold feet. As such it is an excellent circulatory product. It has also gained a good reputation as a painkiller and digestive aid. The main active ingredient is capsaicin—an oily phytochemical. Additionally, it has been used to relieve symptoms of a cold and sore throat.

Garlic

Garlic is excellent for purging candida yeast and parasites from the body. Garlic has so many uses from using it in cooking to it being an excellent product for heart health. It also has antibacterial, anti-fungus and antiviral properties. Other recognized health benefits of Garlic include, acting as an antibiotic and having anti-cholesterol and anti-hypertensive properties.

It is also an antioxidant which protects the body against the effects of free radical damage. Its high sulfur content assists in cell purification.

Allicin is the principle biological active compound which gives Garlic its odor. Be warned. Many so called "odorless" Garlic products have the active compound removed which makes it rather worthless. It can be obtained as a Garlic bulb, in a capsule or in tablet form.

Parsley

Parsley is probably one of the best known herbs as it is used in culinary dishes as well as for medicinal uses. It comes in a variety of different "leaf types", from feather like to curled to flat. The flat leafed variety is most often used for medicinal purposes.

It is used to treat urinary tract infections, indigestion, to relieve the effects of gas and as a digestive aid. Additionally, it is a natural body deodorizer and eradicates bad breath.

Functions of the Digestive System

Basic Function

The basic function of the digestive system is the breakdown and assimilation of foods, primarily carbohydrates, fats and proteins:

- Protein into Amino Acids
- Carbohydrates into Sugar & Starches
- Fats into Fatty Acids

Stomach

Secretes some enzymes and hydrochloric acid (HCl) to break down protein. Within 2-6 hours, all food is emptied into the small intestine.

Small Intestine

Over 90 percent of digestion and absorption takes place here. The acid in the stomach is neutralized and food is mixed with enzymes, bile and pancreatic juices.

Liver

Aids in digestion and detoxification of food impurities and inspects nutrients before allowing them into the bloodstream.

Gallbladder

Stores bile used to break down dietary fat.

Pancreas

Produces digestive juices and helps control blood sugar.

Common Problems Associated With The Digestive System:

- Indigestion
- Heartburn
- Insufficient enzymes
- Stomach ulcers
- Stomach cramps

Lifestyle Suggestions:

- Avoid caffeine, alcohol and soft drinks
- Eat raw fruits and vegetables rich in enzymes
- Avoid overeating
- Eat no later than 2-3 hours before bedtime
- Avoid resting after meals

Interesting Facts:

70-year-old's may produce as little as half the enzymes they produced when they were 20. By age 50, many people will produce only 15 percent of the hydrochloric acid (HCl) they did at age 25, and about a third of all people over the age of 65 secrete almost none

Digestive problems cost the Nation billions each year in medical bills and absence from work.

Supplements for Digestive System Health

For Acid and indigestion:

Papaya

Papaya contains proteolytic enzymes that aid in the digestion of proteins.

Peppermint

Peppermint stimulates the production of digestive fluids. It also eradicates bad breath and helps settle an upset stomach. If purchased in liquid form, then only tiny drops should be applied to water, otherwise it will be too strong.

Activated Charcoal

Absorbs poisons in the digestive tract. Activated Charcoal is one of the best remedies for arresting acute diarrhea, bloating, chemical poisoning, high cholesterol, foul belching and severe gas.

To Support the Liver:

Milk Thistle

This natural support to the liver contains a mixture of bioflavonoids, including silymarin. Milk Thistle strengthens the liver against autointoxication and stimulates protein synthesis in liver cells, which generates DNA and RNA.

For Under Acid Conditions, Heavy Feeling in the Stomach:

Korean Ginseng

Korean Ginseng—also called Panax Ginseng—has been used for over 5,000 years as a preventative tonic to nourish the whole body, especially for stress, fatigue and weak conditions. It grows primarily in China, South Korea and Japan.

Korean Ginseng is considered the strongest form of ginseng. Ginsenoside compounds assist in lowering blood sugar levels, while polysaccharides help to enhance the immune system. Korean Ginseng's antioxidant properties help to stimulate the immune system to help protect the body from various diseases and stress.

Korean Ginseng assists in the production of endorphins which makes a person feel exhilarated. It also has significant sexual health benefits to help improve erectile function, as well as increasing testosterone levels and sperm count.

Enzymes

If you are enzyme deficient (which most people are) due to a lack of enzymes in the food, or the way it is cooked and/or processed, then you can purchase a multi-enzyme product. Make sure though that there are no artificial fillers or additives in it. I have provided a list of enzymes and their function elsewhere in this book.

Functions of the Glandular System

Basic Function

Among their many functions, glands regulate emotions, promote growth, determine sexual identity, control body temperature and assist in the repair of damaged tissue.

Pituitary Gland

About the size of a pea, this gland resides in the brain and is often called the master gland because it secretes hormones that regulate virtually every other gland in the body.

Pineal Gland

The tiny pineal gland (also known as the third eye) is shaped like a pine cone and is located in the center of the brain. It secretes melatonin—a hormone that affects waking and sleep patterns. The production of melatonin is stimulated by darkness and inhibited by light.

When seen under X-rays the pineal gland is often calcified due in part to fluoride in drinking water and toothpaste.

The pineal gland is activated by daylight and controls various body functions in harmony with the hypothalamus gland.

The Hypothalamus Gland

One of the most important functions of the hypothalamus is to link the nervous system to the endocrine system via the pituitary gland (the master gland).

The hypothalamus secretes and synthesizes nerve hormones which in turn secrete or inhibit the secretion of pituitary hormones.

Body temperature is controlled by the hypothalamus, and it is also in charge of directing the body's emotions and feelings, such as: thirst, hunger, sexual desire as well as the biological clock that is responsible for determining the aging process.

Adrenal Glands

Situated atop the kidneys, these glands secrete several hormones. Adrenaline (epinephrine) is well-known: it stimulates the heart, keeps blood pressure normal and raises blood sugar levels. Along with making sex hormones, these glands secrete hormones that help regulate metabolism.

Thyroid Gland

This gland heavily influences growth and the metabolic rate (i.e., the level of activity within the body). That's why the thyroid should be checked when a person is either overweight or underweight. Located at the base of the front of the neck, it influences our motions, intellectual ability and physical vitality, and it was once considered our master gland.

Parathyroid Glands

Acting in concert with the thyroid in controlling the balance of calcium, these four pea-sized structures are attached to the back of the thyroid.

Thymus Gland

Butterfly-shaped and similar to the thyroid, the thymus is high in the chest behind the sternum (breast bone). Formed mostly of lymphatic tissue, it plays a key role in producing the immune system's T -cells (T stands for thymus). T -cells circulate in the blood and lymph to help protect the body from invaders or malignant cells.

Pancreas

This flat, yellow gland is about 5 inches long, residing just below the left side of the rib cage. It has two main functions: 1) to manufacture enzymes that help digest food, and 2) to secrete insulin, a hormone that helps regulate the amount of glucose (a type of sugar) in the blood. Glucose is used for energy.

Ovaries

Located on each side of the lower abdomen of women, these glands regulate the reproductive process through hormone secretions. Ovulation is the release of an egg from an ovary.

Testes

Located outside the body for better temperature control, they manufacture and store spermatozoa. They also produce testosterone, which controls the physical and mental characteristics of a male.

Common Problems Associated With The Glandular System:

- Hormone imbalance
- Emotional stress
- Reproductive troubles
- Hyper/hypo sugar levels

Lifestyle Suggestions:

- Eat regular, wholesome meals.

- Avoid smoking, alcohol and stimulants.
- Exercise regularly.
- Manage your stress.

Interesting Facts

- Every hormone is conveyed through either blood or lymph to stimulate or inhibit the activity of another organ or tissue.
- Prolonged stress can shrivel the thymus and lymph glands and exhaust the adrenals, which tire of trying to keep up with demand.

Supplements for Glandular System Health

Low Blood Sugar:

Licorice Root

Licorice has long been recognized for the natural sweetness of its deep-sinking roots. Next to ginseng, licorice is the most popular herb used in Chinese formulas. It helps support the adrenal glands during periods of stress.

High Blood Sugar—Diabetes:

Nopal

Nopal or Mexican Cactus as it is sometimes called is traditionally used by the Mexicans as a food especially in salads. The nutritional factors in Nopal act in the bowel to prevent fat and excessive sugars from entering the bloodstream. By helping the body maintain balanced blood sugar levels, Nopal aids the body in its battle against obesity. Additionally, it is used as an anti-inflammatory, as a laxative and as a hypoglycemic vehicle for diabetes and gastritis.

Gymnema Sylvestre

Gymnema Sylvestre is a climbing plant which is native to Australia, parts of Africa and central and southern India, and is used in Ayurvedic medicine. It is primarily used for weight management to control appetite and cravings, but has also been used to treat constipation and diabetes.

Chromium

Chromium is a trace mineral essential for proper pancreatic function. It assists in regulating insulin in the body and therefore has an effect on how much energy you get from your food. It helps to reduce food cravings and improves lifespan. It is also important for proper heart function.

Adrenal Exhaustion:

B Complex

B-vitamins are particularly important for the nervous system and are also vital for good digestive function and enzyme reactions that control energy, circulation, hormones and overall health. Since the same amount of each B vitamin is not necessarily needed by the body; this formula is usually balanced to assist B 12 absorption.

Hypothyroidism:

Spirulina

Spirulina is a type of fresh-water blue-green algae composed of approximately 65-71 percent protein making it one of the richest vegetable sources of protein known. These proteins are biologically complete, containing all 9 essential amino acids in their proper ratios.

Much of the protein in spirulina is in the form of biliprotein which has been pre-digested by algae, making it 5 times easier to break down than either meat or soy protein. In fact, the digestibility of spirulina protein is rated 85 percent, compared to approximately 20 percent for beef protein.

This easy to digest type of protein is especially beneficial for those suffering from problems associated with excessive animal protein and refined foods intake-namely those with arthritis, cancer, diabetes, hypoglycemia, obesity, or similar degenerative conditions.

Kelp

Kelp is a brown algae that comes from the sea. It responds to sunlight and takes in minerals and other nutrients from the water. It is an excellent source of iodine. Iodine is needed for proper functioning of the thyroid and pituitary glands.

The thyroid is responsible for maintaining metabolism and body temperature. In fact during stressful periods, the thyroid can work overtime to try and normalize body functions, therefore supplementing with kelp can be very beneficial for boosting energy.

A proper functioning metabolism is also important for maintaining weight control, which can sometimes be a problem when the body is under stress, and a person is susceptible to "binge eat" on comfort foods.

Supplements for Glandular System Health—Female

Menstrual:

Dong Quai

Dong Quai—a member of the celery family—is one of the oldest known herbs, having been used in China, Japan and Korea for over 1,000 years. Known as a women's product, to relieve menopausal symptoms: hot flashes, menstrual disorders such as cramps, irregular menstrual cycles, infrequent periods, premenstrual syndrome (PMS), and menopausal symptoms.

It is suggested that Dong Quai contains compounds that may help reduce pain, dilate blood vessels, and stimulate and relax uterine muscles.

In traditional Chinese medicine (TCM), different parts of the Dong Quai root are used for different actions in the body: the root head is used as an anticoagulant, the main part of the root is used as a tonic, and the tail-end of the root is used to remove blood stagnation. Because it is a balancer of the female hormonal system, it is often called "female's ginseng."

Menopause:

Black Cohosh

Black Cohosh is widely used to treat menopausal symptoms such as hot flashes, night sweats, migraines, mood swings, heart palpitations and dryness. The roots of the plant are used medically and are available as capsules, a liquid extract or tablets.

Pregnancy:

Red Raspberry

This herb is renowned for its nutritional support of the female reproductive system. Red Raspberry is known to nourish and strengthen the uterus. A common backyard fruit bush, Red Raspberry is an excellent herbal source of iron, manganese and niacin. It also contains quantities of vitamins C, A, D, E and B, as well as phosphorus and calcium.

Desire: Infertility:

Maca

Maca, also known as Peruvian Ginseng is used to increase stamina, energy and sexual function in both men and women. In one study, researchers found that Maca may help alleviate sexual dysfunction caused by the use of selective-serotonin re-uptake inhibitors (SSRIs) which are used in the treatment of depression.

Supplements for Glandular System Health—Male

Benign Prostatic Hyperplasia

Saw Palmetto

Saw palmetto is mainly used to treat benign prostatic hyperplasia (BPH). BPH is a male condition which includes frequent urination, difficulty in fulfilling the urge to urinate, dribbling after urination, a weak urinary stream, and finally, waking up several times at night to urinate.

Erectile Dysfunction

Yohimbe

A native to the Congo, Cameroon, Nigeria, and Gabon, Yohimbe is used to prevent depression as it inhibits monoamine oxidase (MAO). Additionally it is used to treat erectile dysfunction either as a single herb, or in combination with other herbs.

Korean Ginseng

Korean Ginseng—also called Panax Ginseng—has been used for over 5,000 years as a preventative tonic to nourish the whole body, especially for stress, fatigue and weak conditions. It grows primarily in China, South Korea and Japan.

Korean Ginseng is considered the strongest form of ginseng. Ginsenoside compounds assist in lowering blood sugar levels, while polysaccharides help to enhance the immune system. Korean Ginseng's antioxidant properties help to stimulate the immune system to help protect the body from various diseases and stress.

Korean Ginseng assists in the production of endorphins which makes a person feel exhilarated. It also has significant sexual health benefits to help improve erectile function, as well as increasing testosterone levels and sperm count.

Functions of the Immune System

Basic Function

The Immune System provides specialized fighting forces that are tailor-made to combat internal invasions, whether they are microbes or toxic chemicals. It also employs "security patrols" that police the body; these are stationed in lymph nodes, openings of the body and other strategic locations.

Inside the body, a trillion highly specialized cells will launch an unending battle against alien organisms. Within minutes the immune system will sense an enemy's presence and send out scavenger cells, which immediately attack the invaders.

Remember that during any war, there are great "expenses" involved. That translates into a greater than normal requirement for better nutrition, and rest to conserve energy.

Bone Marrow

Produces B cells which go on to produce antibodies. These are the foot soldiers of the system. Antibodies neutralize foreign invaders.

Lymph

Is blood serum that has leaked from the bloodstream into the tissue spaces and is recovered by a network of tiny vessels that separate it from the bloodstream. This fluid brings with it tissue toxins and microbes.

Lymph Nodes

Are gathering points throughout the body where lymph travels to unload toxins and microbes for cleansing.

Tonsils

Are lymph tissue in the throat guarding the respiratory and digestive systems.

Thymus

Located behind the breast bone. This central gland of the lymphatic system helps "train" part of the army of B-cells to convert them into T-cells, which are specialized cells to meet a particular enemy.

Spleen

A lymphatic gland under the left ribs, the spleen helps filter the blood and is a pumping aid for lymph fluids throughout the body. It is involved in the production of white blood cells.

Common Problems Associated With The Immune System:

- Viral/bacterial attack
- Fatigue
- Stress
- Cancer
- AIDS

Lifestyle Suggestions:

- Reduce stress.
- Eat lots of fruits and vegetables.
- Eat adequate complete proteins.
- Avoid simple sugars.
- Get adequate sleep and exercise.

Interesting Facts:

- Immunity comes from the word "immunis," a Latin word meaning "safe." In any given year, roughly 50 percent of Americans will catch a cold, and 40 percent will get the flu. 80 percent of all illnesses can be traced to stress.
- Your whole personal immune army weighs about two pounds and consists of about a trillion cells assisted by 100 quintillion antibody molecules.

Supplements for Immune System Health

Bacteria, Virus, Fungus:

Garlic

This popular herb offers a boost to the immune system with its antibacterial, antifungal and antiviral properties.

Garlic has many uses:

- Anti-biotic—natural penicillin
- Arteriosclerosis
- Arthritis
- Asthma
- Blood poisoning
- High blood pressure

- Anti-viral
- Anti-bacterial
- Destroys many types of parasites
- For respiratory conditions use with Mullein or Lobelia
- As a decongestant / expectorant use with Lobelia
- For bacterial infection use with Golden Seal, Echinacea, Pau d'Arco
- For viral infection use with colloidal silver
- For yeast infections use with Pau d'Arco
- For swollen lymph nodes use with Lobelia and Mullein
- For parasites use with Pumpkin Seeds and Black Walnut

Colloidal Silver

Colloidal silver has many uses and has been found to be effective against many surface and internal micro-organisms, viruses, protozoa, amoeba, fungi, parasites and yeasts. It works by in-activating the enzyme that is responsible for the multiplication of many of these invaders.

There are many different colloidal silver products on the market. You need to source one that contains 99.9 percent pure silver, without any additives, apart from purified water.

Echinacea

Echinacea contains polysaccharides that stimulate the production of phagocytes (cells that engulf and consume foreign matter) and activate T-lymphocytes, macrophages and natural killer cells. Taken at the earliest sign of a cold or infection, Echinacea may help cut recovery time considerably.

Olive Leaf Extract

Olive Leaf Extract supports normal blood pressure and cholesterol levels and strengthens the immune system against viral and bacterial attacks.

Una de Gato (Cats Claw)

- The bark of a vine from South America. Una de Gato provides beneficial alkaloids to stimulate the immune system. It is also used for the following:
- As a cancer therapy to reduce the side effects of chemotherapy.
- As an anti-inflammatory for all types of arthritis

- As a bowel and stomach protector and cleanser, and to treat ulcerative colitis as well as stomach ulcers.
- To treat a variety of bowel problems including, but not limited to: Crohn's disease, diverticulitis and irritable bowel syndrome (IBS).
- An excellent general body tonic to tone and protect all body systems.
- It is usually taken in capsule form.

Elderberry

One of the oldest known herbs. It works in the respiratory and immune body systems, and is usually used to counter the effects of colds, flu, congestion, sore throat and inflammation.

Zinc Lozenges

Zinc is often combined with Echinacea and Licorice Root (as a natural sweetener) to treat the effects of a sore throat or other mouth infections. It also supplies excellent immune system support.

When buying this type of product, make sure there are no artificial fillers or artificial sugar coatings which would be used as a sweetener.

Pau D'Arco

Pau D'Arco is native to South America. It contains a chemical called lapachol, which may provide nutritional support to the immune system. It is commonly used against many conditions of unwanted growth, including fungus, yeast and tumors as well as fungal infections. Historically, it has also been used to remedy the side effects of some antibiotics.

It is available as a capsule, tablet or as a lotion.

Bifidophilus

A probiotic supplement. Bifidophilus products contain living organisms from various strains of "friendly" bacteria to help replace depleted bacteria in the colon. They are necessary for proper immune function, and to help balance the digestive system.

Probiotics are beneficial after taking a course of antibiotics. Antibiotics not only kill foreign invaders, but they kill "friendly" bacteria too.

Vitamin C

The common cold and flu are viral infections. If you increase your intake of vitamin C by taking a high dose supplement then your cold will clear up much quicker. Vitamin C is also water soluble so it is easily depleted in the body.

Compromised Immune System:

Una de Gato (Cats Claw)

The bark of a vine from South America. Una de Gato provides beneficial alkaloids to stimulate the immune system. It is also used for the following:

- As a cancer therapy to reduce the side effects of chemotherapy.
- As an anti-inflammatory for all types of arthritis.
- As a bowel and stomach protector and cleanser, and to treat ulcerative colitis as well as stomach ulcers.
- To treat a variety of bowel problems including, but not limited to: Crohn's disease, diverticulitis and irritable bowel syndrome (IBS).
- An excellent general body tonic to tone and protect all body systems.
- It is usually taken in capsule form.

Free Radical Damage:

Proanthocyanidins

Often sold under the trade name Pycnogenol. Proanthocyanidins are powerful antioxidants obtained from grape seed and pine bark. They help prevent cell damage by quenching oxidative free radicals. This combination of antioxidant nutrients has been shown to be many times more powerful than vitamin C or E. Proanthocyanidins also improve the integrity of collagen fibers, strengthening tissues in the skin, blood vessels, muscles, cartilage and other connective tissues.

Any Other Antioxidants

There are antioxidant vitamins: vitamins A, C and E, and Beta Carotene, antioxidant minerals: selenium and zinc, and antioxidant herbs: garlic, ginkgo biloba and many others have antioxidant properties. All provide protection against free radical damage. Unless there are other health issues where specific herbal products may be required, which would provide some antioxidant protection, the usual way to help protect the body against the effects of free radical damage is to take an antioxidant vitamin and mineral supplement.

Functions of the Intestinal System

Basic Function

The intestines comprise the small intestine, large intestine and the rectum. The small intestine is approximately 20 feet long and about one inch in diameter. Its function is to absorb the nutrients from food through velvety tissue called villi.

The large intestine (or colon) is approximately five feet long and approximately three inches in diameter. Water is absorbed from waste which then creates a stool. The stool enters the rectum where nerves impulses create the urge to eliminate it.

Small Intestine

Over 90 percent of digestion and absorption takes place here. The acid of the stomach is neutralized, and food is mixed with enzymes, bile and pancreatic juices. The small intestine is usually considered part of the digestive system, since almost all nutrients are processed and absorbed by the time the residue of a meal reaches the large intestine.

Large Intestine

Also called the colon or lower bowel. It is divided into three parts: ascending (from the end of the small intestine near the appendix, up the abdominal cavity on the right side); transverse (crossing just under the ribs in front of the stomach); and descending (down the left side to the rectum). Acting as a "compactor," the large intestine is aided by the presence and pressure of undigested fiber. This compacting action tends to cleanse the inner walls of the intestine, and during this squeezing, water is withdrawn, with a few ounces left to help prevent constipation.

The Ileocecal Valve

Is a muscle that opens to allow food waste to pass to the large intestine and then closes to prevent any from traveling back in the wrong direction. With different bacteria present in these areas, this valve keeps them in the right places.

The Appendix

Is lymph tissue that guard against infection. When it is weakened, it may become infected, swell or burst, endangering life.

The Rectum

The last five inches of the colon, ends with the anus, a powerful muscle which controls evacuation.

Common Problems Associated With The Intestinal System:

- Constipation/diarrhea
- Hemorrhoids
- Diverticulitis
- Colitis
- Crohn's disease
- Irritable bowel syndrome

Lifestyle Suggestions:

- Make sure you get adequate fiber in your diet
- Exercising can stimulate the intestinal system to work properly
- Avoid high fat foods
- Avoid foods containing excessive amounts of sugar
- Eat plenty of fresh fruits and vegetables

Interesting Fact:

- You may house 400 species and 100 trillion bacteria in your colon. Some of them synthesize vitamin K, B12 and biotin. Others (Friendly Flora) neutralize toxins and help control dangerous bacteria.

Supplements for Intestinal System Health

Diarrhea:

Bentonite (montmorillonite) Clay

Bentonite clay is very quick acting as it has the ability to bind the stools together. It does this by binding irritants in the gastrointestinal tract. One option is to combine the bentonite clay with a small quantity of applesauce to make the clay more palatable. Applesauce contains pectin—another binding agent. Incidentally pectin is also used in jam making to make the fruit "set".

Activated Charcoal

Charcoal is highly absorbent. Activated Charcoal can help in cases of poisoning or severe diarrhea as it absorbs irritants and toxins in the digestive tract. It may also help lower cholesterol levels as well as relieving the effects of foul belching and severe smelly gas. An alternative to activated charcoal is to use bentonite clay.

Constipation:

Psyllium

An excellent source of dietary fiber. Psyllium is gluten free and is therefore a useful fiber source for those suffering from celiac disease or gluten intolerance.

It expands dramatically from the size of the original seeds and it is therefore essential to drink plenty of water with this product.

Psyllium absorbs toxins from the intestinal tract and binds them to fecal matter for elimination.

As it is a bulking agent, it often gives a feeling of fullness and discourages a person from over eating.

One of the main causes of constipation is a lack of fiber in the diet.

Magnesium

This essential mineral can act as a laxative for a spastic colon (cramping and/or explosive bowel movement, sometimes caused by stress). Some over-the-counter laxatives contain magnesium. It is often combined with calcium to aid the structural system as well as helping relax the nervous system.

B Complex

Where spastic constipation is stress related, a B Complex vitamin supplement may be required along with vitamin C. B vitamins and vitamin C are water soluble and are easily depleted when the body is under stress. They are often referred to as the stress vitamins. Note. All the B vitamins work together so it is usually preferable to take a B Complex supplement and then top-up with individual B vitamins if required.

Parasites:

Black Walnut

Traditionally used as a nutritional aid for the intestinal system, Black Walnut has the same laxative action as Cascara Sagrada, but it works more gently. Due to its astringent qualities, Black Walnut has the power to assist the body in protecting itself from harmful agents such as parasitic worms. It also has a high iodine content, which is good for energy as it supports thyroid function.

Bifidophilus

A probiotic supplement. Bifidophilus products contain living organisms from various strains of "friendly" bacteria to help replace depleted bacteria in the colon. They are necessary for proper immune function, and to help balance the digestive system.

Probiotics are very beneficial after taking a course of antibiotics. Antibiotics not only kill foreign invaders, but they kill "friendly" bacteria too.

Functions of the Nervous System

Basic Function

The basic function of the nervous system is to trigger and monitor all communication process in the body.

While the brain is the master controller, the nervous system also has local control points. For example, a burn reflex travels to and from the spinal cord so you withdraw your hand before your brain knows what happened.

There are three types of neurons: sensory neurons, which receive stimuli and carry impulses to the central nervous system (CNS); inter-neurons, which connect two or more neurons; and motor-neurons, which carry impulses away from the CNS to muscles or glands.

Impulses travel from one nerve cell to another across a synapse with the help of chemical transmitters. Among these are acetylcholine, norepinephrine and serotonin.

Neuron

A nerve cell that includes receiving and transmitting arms that link it to billions of nerve cells throughout the body.

Neurotransmitter

One of several types of chemical messengers.

Brain

As master controller (and weighing an average of three pounds), it uses 20 percent of the body's total energy supply to power an estimated 10 billion brain cells.

Central Nervous System

The brain and spinal cord

Peripheral Nervous System

A network of nerves branching out from the spinal cord that go throughout the body.

Common Problems Associated With The Nervous System:

- Headaches
- Insomnia
- Nervous disorders and memory loss
- Depression

Lifestyle Suggestions:

- Eat regular, wholesome meals.
- Avoid smoking, alcohol and stimulants.
- Exercise regularly.
- Manage your stress.
- Eat lots of green, leafy vegetables, fruits, whole grains and nuts.

Interesting Facts:

- Some nerve fibers can conduct nerve impulses as fast as 200 yards per second.
- Scientists are investigating evidence that dead nerve cells can be replaced by the body, a process once thought to be impossible.
- Prescriptions for antidepressants have increased over 100 percent in the last five years.
- To combat anxiety, a daily walk may be as effective as tranquilizers.

Supplements for Nervous System Health

Stress:

B Complex and Vitamin C

When the body is under stress, a B Complex vitamin supplement may be required along with vitamin C. B vitamins and vitamin C are water soluble and are easily depleted from the body, especially during stressful times. All the B vitamins work together so it is usually preferable to take a B Complex supplement and then top-up with individual B vitamins if required. The B vitamins and vitamin C are often referred to as the stress vitamins.

Depression:

St. John's Wort

This popular herb has gained national attention for its ability to alleviate mild to moderate depression. It contains an active constituent, hypericin, which appears to prolong the activity of serotonin (a neurotransmitter) in the brain. St. John's Wort may also lengthen the performance of dopamine and nor-epinephrine, two brain chemicals that are linked to depression. In Europe, many doctors prescribe this herb instead of prescription antidepressant drugs.

Note! You can find further details on Stress and Depression by reading my Book "*An Easy Way to Understand Stress and Depression*", which is available from the Kindle Store, or there is a download printable version available at www.wisdomforlifemedia.com.

Mind, Memory Loss, Poor Memory:

Ginkgo Biloba

Ginkgo Biloba promotes increased circulation. It also dilates blood vessels and bronchioles to improve circulation and oxygenation of cells. It also has scientifically proven nervous-system benefits in addition to improving memory function.

Huperzine A

Derived from Chinese Club Moss, Huperzine A was shown in a Chinese study in 1999 to enhance memory and learning abilities in a group of adolescent students.

The Cochrane Database of Systematic Reviews published a 2008 research review which showed that Huperzine A was of benefit to individuals suffering from Alzheimer's disease.

Functions of the Respiratory System

Basic Function

The basic function of the respiratory system is to supply the body with oxygen and eliminate its by-product, carbon dioxide.

Fresh air is literally sucked into the body when the diaphragm muscle pulls down inside the chest cavity.

Traveling down the throat into the bronchial tubes, air branches out into the lungs and finally into 300 million tiny alveoli sacs. There, blood flowing close to the inner surface of the lungs exchanges fresh air with carbon dioxide and other waste gases, which are exhaled. Deep breathing makes it all happen more efficiently.

All along these air passages are millions of cilia, about 200 per cell, which help carry foreign particles and toxic mucus out of the lungs, throat and nasal cavities. Cilia move these particles in only one direction, unless they (the cilia) are poisoned by toxins like smoke. For those irritants that remain, immune cells are stationed in the area to engulf and dissolve these small intruders.

Mucus exuded by surface tissues of the respiratory and digestive tract keep respiratory tissues from dehydrating and cracking, in addition, they also have an antiseptic action.

When the body is too toxic, this waste spills over into other areas like the mucus of the respiratory system. This can cause irritation and swelling, and becomes a breeding ground for millions of unwelcome bacteria and viruses.

Sinuses

Here air is both warmed and moisturized for more efficient transfer of gases in the lungs.

Larynx

Air flows past the larynx (voice box) and into the bronchi on its way to the lungs.

Trachea

Also known as the windpipe, it leads to the bronchi.

Bronchi

The trachea leads into these, which subdivide into smaller and smaller passageways, the bronchioles.

Lungs

Within the lungs' air sacs, oxygen trades places with carbon dioxide or other gases that the body considers waste.

Diaphragm

This acts as the body's bellows to push and pull the air you breathe.

Common Problems Associated With The Respiratory System:

- Asthma
- Hay fever
- Coughs
- Bronchitis

Lifestyle Suggestions:

- Do not smoke
- Avoid inhaling other people's smoke
- Make sure your digestive system is working properly
- Make sure your immune system is not compromised
- Eat plenty of fresh fruits and vegetables
- Get plenty of exercise
- Make sure you get adequate rest and sleep

Interesting Facts:

- The total respiratory surface is 25-50 times the surface area of your entire body.
- Non-smokers who are in close proximity to smokers raise their risk for lung cancer by 30 percent.
- Non-smokers in heavy traffic may breathe as many airborne free radicals as a pack-a-day smoker.

Supplements for Respiratory System Health

Deficient Mucus (yellow & Thick), With a Dry Irritated Cough:

Mullein

Mullein has both mucilant and astringent properties. Its powerful healing abilities make it useful for healing weak lung tissue and chronic respiratory congestion. It has proven expectorant action that likely arises from saponin compounds in the plant. Scientific studies suggest that the mucilage in Mullein protects mucous membranes, preventing cell invasion by viral allergens.

Excess Mucus (white, clear or watery mucus):

Fenugreek

Fenugreek is a respiratory system herb which assists in expelling mucous, phlegm and infections from the lungs, and toxic waste through the lymphatic system. In addition, Fenugreek is able to dissolve a hardened build up of mucous which can then be eliminated.

Garlic

A powerful, aromatic herb, Garlic aids decongestion and expectoration. Garlic works especially well on lung congestion. It has known antibacterial and antiviral properties.

Echinacea

There are various strains of Echinacea. It is used to support the immune system and is involved in the production of white blood cells, which assists the body to fight infection. Echinacea purges toxins from the blood and enhances lymphatic drainage.

Golden Seal

Golden seal has infection-fighting abilities and anti-inflammatory properties, especially in the mucus membranes. It is sometimes combined with Echinacea and Garlic to make a really powerful treatment for colds, flu and to treat other infections.

Asthma—caused by anxiety or stress:

Lobelia

Lobelia has a lengthy history of use as an herbal remedy for respiratory conditions such as asthma, bronchitis, pneumonia, and cough. Traditionally, Native Americans smoked Lobelia as a treatment for asthma. Today, some herbalists use Lobelia to help clear mucus from the respiratory tract, including the throat, lungs, and bronchial tubes. Additionally, Lobelia is used as part of a comprehensive treatment plan for asthma.

Asthma—due to a history of hay fever or respiratory allergies:

Alfalfa

Alfalfa is a grass which contains all the essential amino acids as well as being rich in trace minerals and enzymes. It is frequently taken to lessen the effects of hay fever allergies.

As it is a good source of fiber, it is useful for detoxifying the body in addition to improving liver health.

Methyl Sulfonyl Methane (MSM)

Methyl Sulfonyl Methane is a sulfur dietary supplement that starts life in the sea. Plankton in the sea release sulfur compounds which rise into the atmosphere where ultra violet light converts them into MSM and DMSO (dimethyl sulfoxide)—a precursor to MSM.

MSM and DMSO return to earth attached to rain droplets. MSM is found in grains, vegetables, fruits, meat and poultry.

MSM is an organic form of sulfur that is found in living tissues. MSM is the only dietary supplement that relieves allergies and arthritic conditions at the same time. In the structural system it is an excellent treatment for arthritis, muscle pains and bursitis. Additionally it supports connective tissue such as ligaments, tendons, and muscle.

Sulfur is an important element in maintaining good health. But it is lacking in the Western diet. Therefore it would be worth considering as a preventative product.

Proanthocyanidins

Often sold under the trade name Pycnogenol. Proanthocyanidins are powerful antioxidants obtained from grape seed and pine bark. They help prevent cell damage by quenching oxidative free radicals. This combination of antioxidant nutrients has been shown to be many times more powerful than vitamin C or E. Proanthocyanidins also improve the integrity of collagen fibers, strengthening tissues in the skin, blood vessels, muscles, cartilage and other connective tissues.

Alcohol Withdrawal:

Kudzu / St John's Wort

Historically Asian-Healers have used Kudzu to treat colds, flu, high blood pressure, allergies and many other ailments.

More recently, Chinese-Healers have used Kudzu to treat people who have an alcohol dependency. It has also been used with St John's Wort to treat the depressive effects of alcohol withdrawal. Kudzu is available in capsules, tablets, and dried root.

Stopping Smoking:

Lobelia / St John's Wort

Lobelia is used in a smoking prevention regime due to one of its active ingredients—lobeline which reduces the effects of nicotine in the body; especially the release of dopamine. Dopamine plays many important functions in the brain—especially with regard to drug addiction.

Lobelia is sometimes combined with St John's Wort to reduce the depressive and stress effects when a person is trying to give us smoking.

The two herbs provide a cleansing and detoxifying action, in addition to helping clear "tar" from the lungs—one of the health consequences of smoking.

Functions of the Skeletal System

Basic Function

The basic function of the skeleton is to provide support and protection for the body. The skeletal structure is so important that without it, you would end up in a heap on the floor.

The skeleton comprises all the bones in the body as well as some tissues including cartilage, ligaments and tendons that connect them.

In addition, the skeleton provides protection for internal organs: the heart, lungs, brain, eyes and spinal cord.

While teeth are considered part of the skeletal system, they are not made of bone. They are made of enamel and dentine. Enamel is by far the strongest substance in the human body.

Bones

Along with providing a strong foundation to support-or protect-other body parts, the body's 206 bones are living structures that manufacture new blood cells within the marrow. Minerals packed in protein sacs are "glued" together to make healthy bones stronger than iron. Physical activity stimulates the bones to maintain their strength. Bones provide a storehouse for minerals that can be withdrawn in emergencies.

Muscles

Attached to the bones are ligaments that hold bones together and tendons that connect bones to a total of 620 muscles. In addition to moving the body, they produce heat, squeeze blood into isolated tissues, maintain posture and, when exercised, increase endorphin hormones, which results in a feeling of well-being. Muscle tissue surrounds arteries so blood pressure can be increased where tissue nutrients are most needed.

Skin

The skin is the largest organ of the body—and the most exposed. It is a supple, elastic tissue that conserves heat and moisture. It is the first organ to respond to pain or touch. Skin also functions as a cooling system and helps regulate internal body temperature. Skin helps eliminate toxic matter through perspiration and reabsorbs its own surface oils irradiated by the sun in order to make vitamin D.

Hair

Hair follicles can be found almost everywhere in the skin. These are oiled from embedded sebaceous glands, which keep the skin supple and waterproof. Hair is made of keratin protein and helps control body temperature. The root is the only living part and appears to draw toxic metals out of the blood, encapsulating them in dead hair cells that are pushed out of the skin. While hair also protects the body, a nerve attached to each follicle increases the body's sensitivity to touch.

Common Problems Associated With The Skeletal System:

- Arthritis
- Osteoporosis
- Muscle cramps
- Poor posture

Lifestyle Suggestions:

- Eat regular, balanced meals.
- Get adequate sources of calcium.
- Perform weight-bearing exercises, including walking.
- Chew fibrous fruits and vegetables for strong teeth.
- Practice oral hygiene.

Interesting Facts:

- There are 100,000 strands of hair on the average head.
- Muscle tissue comprises about 40 percent of your body weight.
- Bedridden patients have been known to lose as much as one percent of their inner bone per week.

Supplements for Skeletal System Health

Joint Inflammation:

Alfalfa

Alfalfa is a grass which contains all the essential amino acids as well as being rich in trace minerals and enzymes. It is used to reduce joint inflammation in humans as well as in animals—especially horses.

Methyl Sulfonyl Methane (MSM)

Methyl Sulfonyl Methane is a sulfur dietary supplement that starts life in the sea. Plankton in the sea release sulfur compounds which rise into the atmosphere where ultra violet light converts them into MSM and DMSO (dimethyl sulfoxide)—a precursor to MSM.

MSM and DMSO return to earth attached to rain droplets. MSM is found in grains, vegetables, fruits, meat and poultry.

MSM is an organic form of sulfur that is found in living tissues. MSM is the only dietary supplement that relieves allergies and arthritic conditions at the same time. In the skeletal system it is an excellent treatment for arthritis, muscle pains and bursitis. Additionally it supports connective tissue such as ligaments, tendons, and muscle.

Sulfur is an important element in maintaining good health. But it is lacking in the Western diet. Therefore it would be worth considering as a preventative product.

Glucosamine

Glucosamine is a building block of cartilage. As such, it helps relieve arthritic symptoms and restore cartilage health. By supplementing with glucosamine, it is possible to strengthen and rebuild cartilage throughout the body

Chondroitin

Chondroitin attracts fluid into the joints, where it acts as a shock absorber during impact. This fluid also brings vital nutrients to the cartilage. Chondroitin protects the cartilage from premature disintegration.

It is available in supplement form with glucosamine. Additionally, it can also be obtained as a glucosamine, chondroitin and MSM supplement.

Skin Problems:

Evening Primrose Oil

Evening Primrose Oil assists the body in producing prostaglandins. Evening Primrose Oil provides omega-6 essential fatty acids that help with eczema and brittle nails.

Eczema & Psoriasis:

Pau D'Arco Lotion

Herbalists have long used Pau d'Arco to enhance and fortify the human immune system. Pau d'Arco Lotion is specially formulated for topical use on rashes on hands, arms and face. The emollient properties of Pau d'Arco leave skin feeling smooth and supple.

Acne:

Tea Tree Oil

A native of Australia. Tea Tree Oil has many uses. It is highly prized for its antiseptic and anti-bacterial benefits. It is used to treat acne, athlete's foot, abscesses, boils, dandruff and Pyorrhea. It is also used to sterilize cuts,

Bone Health and Hair, Skin and Nails:

Horsetail

This herb has diuretic properties and can help with some kidney conditions. It is particularly effective for healing when blood is present in the urine. Horsetail also has astringent properties and as such, is used for bed-wetting in children and incontinence in Adults.

Horsetail is rich in silica, which helps to soothe and strengthen connective tissue. Silica is required for bone and cartilage formation, as well as assisting the body in absorbing and utilizing calcium. Calcium is needed for repairing fractures and treating bone diseases, including rickets and osteoporosis. Horsetail is used to strengthen bones, teeth, nails and hair. The improved cartilage helps to lessen inflammation and combat joint pain, arthritis, gout, muscle cramps, hemorrhoids, spasms and rheumatism.

The silica content in Horsetail also promotes the growth of collagen, which is a protein found in connective tissue, Collagen assists in improving skin health and tone.

Functions of the Urinary System

Basic Function

After the body has adsorbed nutrients from the food, waste products are created which circulate in the blood and in the colon. The urinary system works in harmony with the lungs, skin, and intestines—all of which also excrete wastes—to keep the chemicals and water in the body balanced.

Urea is one type of waste the urinary system removes. Urea is created when certain proteins from meat and poultry and specific vegetables are broken down in the body. This waste material is then carried through the bloodstream to the kidneys for filtration.

More than 2 million filters in the kidneys separate toxic elements and excessive amounts of nutrients that cannot be stored or utilized (including water) from the blood.

The kidneys adjust the blood's pH by maintaining the proper sodium/potassium balance necessary for each cell to make energy. These organs can even secrete hormones to help regulate the body.

After the kidneys extract just enough water to keep the body healthy, urine flows down a ureter (tube) into the bladder for storage. From there, it empties through another tube (urethra) to the outside.

Kidneys

Two kidneys reside behind the stomach, nestled in a protective cushion of fat. When they are inflamed, the kidneys ache and some people mistake this for a backache. But this backache can occur during any severe battle the body is waging in which lots of toxins are being processed and overloading the kidneys' ability to filter them out, thus actually tiring and poisoning the kidneys themselves.

Ureter

Attached to the bottom of each kidney, these tubes carry urine into the bladder.

Bladder

Urine is stored here. After it builds up, nerves signal the brain that it's time to be emptied. Holding urine too long in the bladder can encourage bacterial growth or cause chemical irritation.

Common Problems Associated With The Urinary System:

- Bladder/kidney infection
- Kidney stones
- Incontinence
- Cystitis
- Pain and irritation

Lifestyle Suggestions:

- Drink 64 oz. of water daily.
- Drink unsweetened cranberry juice.
- Eat lots of fruits and vegetables.
- Practice personal hygiene.

What Your Kidneys Do For You:

- Help regulate blood pressure
- Adjust the amount of fluid in the body.
- Contribute to a proper pH balance vital for normal chemical reactions throughout the body. They re-absorb 90 percent of the filtered materials as a conservation measure.
- Remove blood toxins and non-storable excess nutrients or water.
- Help maintain proper sodium/potassium balance for more energy production.

Interesting Facts:

- The kidneys recycle about 45 gallons of blood every day.
- 25 percent of your blood is being filtered in the kidneys at all times.
- Inside the kidneys are 2.4 million nephron filters requiring 50 miles of tiny capillaries and tubules.

Supplements for Urinary System Health

Irritated & Inflamed Urinary Tract:

Uva Ursi

Uva Ursi is used to treat cystitis—inflammation of the urinary tract. The main component of Uva Ursi is arbutin. Arbutin is absorbed in the stomach where it is converted into a substance with antimicrobial, astringent and antimicrobial properties.

Arbutin's main purpose is to soothe irritation and reduce inflammation during urination, as well as to fight infections in the urinary tract.

It is important for the urine to be alkaline for Uva Ursi to work properly. The acid / alkaline balance (pH) can be determined by using a litmus paper test strip. If the urine is too acidic then it can be brought to an alkaline state by the use of alkalizing agents such as calcium, magnesium supplements, chlorophyll in liquid form (chlorophyll is derived from alfalfa), and by eating alkalizing foods such as tomatoes, and the majority of fruits and vegetables. This is by no means a complete list. Note. While most citrus fruits are acidic, when they have been digested they are alkaline forming.

Acidic foods to avoid would be mainly beef, pork, lamb, butter, peanut butter, and many more. There are some excellent acid / alkaline food lists available on the Internet. Just type "acid alkaline food lists" into your search engine.

Marshmallow

This mucilant soothes the kidneys when they are irritated or inflamed. Marshmallow contains volatile oils and tannins that are responsible for its diuretic actions. It is especially helpful in passing kidney stones.

Urinary Tract Infections:

Cranberry / Buchu

Cranberry main purpose is to treat bacterial infections in the bladder. It is often combined with Buchu herb.

When used together, these two herbs have anti-inflammatory, diuretic and antiseptic properties. Scientific studies show that Cranberry makes the urinary tract inhospitable to bacteria, lessening the risk of urinary tract infections. Buchu acts as a diuretic and improves digestion. This product works best in acidic urine conditions.

Golden Seal

Golden seal has infection-fighting abilities and anti-inflammatory properties, and can be used as an alternative to Cranberry if required.

Kidney Weakness:

Potassium

Potassium controls the balance of fluids in the body. In the urinary system it is used to treat water retention and various urinary problems. Consider taking a potassium supplement where there is a potassium deficiency due to excess flushing caused by urinary tract infections.

Horsetail

This herb has diuretic properties and can help with some kidney conditions. It is particularly effective for healing when blood is present in the urine. Horsetail also has astringent properties and as such, is used for bed-wetting in children and incontinence in Adults.

Horsetail is rich in silica, which helps to soothe and strengthen connective tissue. Silica is required for bone and cartilage formation, as well as assisting the body in absorbing and utilizing calcium. Calcium is required for repairing fractures and treating bone diseases, including rickets and osteoporosis. Horsetail is used to strengthen bones, teeth, nails and hair. The improved cartilage helps to lessen inflammation and combat joint pain, arthritis, gout, muscle cramps, hemorrhoids, spasms and rheumatism.

The silica content in Horsetail also promotes the growth of collagen, which is a protein found in connective tissue, Collagen assists in improving skin health and tone.

Weight Loss

An overweight and imbalanced body is often linked. Thousands of people die annually from all kinds of different weight related illnesses which are often connected to poor diet and a compromised lifestyle. A recent nationwide survey found the more overweight a person is, the higher the incidence of major health problems.

Here are some of the illnesses that people die from each year, which are all weight related.

- Arteriosclerosis
- Cancer
- Coronary heart disease
- Gallbladder disease
- Hypertension
- Stroke
- Type 11 diabetes

The following supplements could help in a weight loss program.

Multivitamin and Mineral

A good quality multivitamin and mineral supplement will ensure that you do not have a dietary shortfall. I have discussed multivitamins and minerals and their benefits elsewhere in this book. You can then add some of the items listed below, all of which are helpful in achieving weight loss.

B vitamins

B vitamins are intimately linked to weight loss. B3 and B6 assist in supplying fuel to cells which is then converted to energy. Vitamin B6 together with zinc is needed for the production of pancreatic enzymes which are produced by the pancreas to digest proteins, carbohydrates, and fats in the small intestine. This ensures that food is digested properly, rather than it being stored as fat.

Vitamins B2, B3 and B6 are needed for the production of thyroid hormones. Any deficiencies will result in an inadequate thyroid gland function which will affect body metabolism.

Vitamin B3 is a component of the glucose tolerance factor (GTF) which is involved each time blood sugar levels rise. Vitamin B5 is involved in energy production and helps to control fat metabolism.

As I have mentioned elsewhere in this book, the B vitamins work together, so it is beneficial to take a good quality, natural B Complex supplement.

Excessive Sugar Consumption:

This would include high blood sugar, indications of diabetes and a high sugar diet.

Chromium

This mineral has been well researched in relation to weight loss. It is necessary for the metabolism of sugar and if it is lacking, then insulin is less effective in controlling blood sugar levels. If this happens, then it is harder to burn off food as fuel and it is more likely that the body will store it as fat. Chromium also helps to control fat levels and cholesterol circulating in the blood.

Zinc

This is an important antioxidant mineral in appetite control. A deficiency can cause a loss of taste and smell, creating a need for stronger tasting foods (which tend to be sweeter, saltier and more fattening!) Zinc also functions with vitamins A and E to manufacture the thyroid hormones.

Co-Enzyme Q10

Co-Enzyme Q10 (Co-Q10) is necessary for energy production. The body manufactures Co-Q10 itself and it is found in every cell of the body. As a person ages, less of it is produced so there could be a deficiency which will result in a reduction of energy. Additionally, if a person takes a statin drug to reduce cholesterol, then this person will be very deficient as statins destroy Co-Q10. Co-Q10 is intimately linked to heart health, it also helps reduces hypertension (high blood pressure) and deficiencies of the immune system.

Garcinia Cambogia

Garcinia cambogia is a tropical fruit which contains HCA (hydroxy-citric acid), which stimulates the body to burn carbohydrates as energy rather than storing them as fat. HCA acts as an appetite suppressant which reduces the intake of food, thus reducing fat and cholesterol formation.

Nopal

Nopal or Mexican Cactus as it is sometimes called is traditionally used by the Mexicans as a food especially in salads. The nutritional factors in Nopal act in the bowel to prevent fat and excessive sugars from entering the bloodstream. By helping the body maintain balanced blood sugar levels, Nopal aids the body in its battle against obesity. Additionally, it is used as an anti-inflammatory, as a laxative and as a hypoglycemic vehicle for diabetes and gastritis.

Meal Replacement – Snacks and Appetite:

Spirulina

Spirulina is a type of fresh-water blue-green algae composed of approximately 65-71 percent protein making it one of the richest vegetable sources of protein known. These proteins are biologically complete, containing all 9 essential amino acids in their proper ratios.

Much of spirulina's protein is in the form of biliprotein which has been pre-digested by algae, making it 5 times easier to break down than either meat or soy protein. In fact, the digestibility of spirulina protein is rated 85 percent, compared to approximately 20 percent for beef protein.

This easy to digest type of protein is especially beneficial for those suffering from problems associated with excessive animal protein and refined foods intake-namely those with arthritis, cancer, diabetes, hypoglycemia, obesity, or similar degenerative conditions.

It is useful in a weight loss program, as it is a complete source of protein, it suppresses the appetite by giving a feeling of fullness, and the person is less likely to snack on unsuitable foods.

Metabolism:

CLA

CLA, or conjugated linoleic acid, is a mixture of essential fatty acids that are important for maintaining healthy body functions.

CLA helps to sustain lean muscle mass as well as enhancing the burning of fat, which makes it a useful product in a weight-loss regime.

Hoodia Gordonii

Hoodia Gordonii is actually a succulent plant that grows in the semi-deserts of South Africa, Botswana, Namibia, and Angola. It grows in clumps of green upright stems which after five years produce a pale purple flower, at which time the plant can be harvested.

Interestingly, there are said to be more than 13 varieties of hoodia. But only Hoodia Gordonii has so far been identified to contain an active ingredient, a steroidal glycoside that has been named "p57".

Much of the marketing hype stems from stories of San Bushmen who live in the Kalahari Desert. These bushmen are said to have taken hoodia for thousands of years to stave off hunger pangs and thirst whilst on long hunting trips. Today Hoodia Gordonii is sold as a weight loss product and is available as a capsule, powder, and tea or liquid.

Morinda Citrifolia (Noni)

A native of the Polynesian Islands—Tahiti and Hawaii—Morinda Citrifolia (Noni) has been used by the Polynesians for over 2,000 years for a variety of treatments including: bacterial, viral, fungal, and tumors. Additionally it has been used as a hypotensive, for anti-inflammatory conditions, and to support the immune system. Further uses include: boosting metabolism in a weight management program.

Morinda is available in capsules and also as a liquid. In liquid form the raw Morinda has a very bitter taste, so it is often sweetened with natural licorice or glycerin.

Fiber and Exercise:

No weight loss program would be complete without mentioning fiber intake, exercise and getting adequate rest and sleep.

I have mentioned fiber quite a lot in this book. To recap: it is important to clear toxins out of the colon and to purge intestinal parasites. I mentioned in my book "*An Easy Way to Understand Parasites, Worms, Candida and Detoxing*", (available on Amazon.com or from www.wisdomforlifemedia.com) that many people have experienced a weight loss of several pounds by doing a detox program. This extra weight was all compacted toxic matter that had resided in the colon—in some cases for many years.

Exercise is important for circulatory system health as well as for stimulating the immune system. These two systems are linked to all the other body systems and they all work in harmony with one another. If one of these systems is misfiring, then the whole body will be out of balance, which can lead to all kinds of health conditions.

Not only that—exercise is good for you. But you must choose an exercise program that you will enjoy doing. If it becomes a chore then you will soon get bored with it, and give it up.

My chosen exercise is bike riding. I usually go for an hour each day. Because it is really hot and humid in the summertime where we live, I usually go either early in the morning or late in the evening.

So I don't get bored, I have four different routes to choose from. My wife enjoys bike riding too, as well as walking and playing tennis. We both do our exercise program seven day per week, unless we are traveling.

If you do a vigorous exercise regime or play sports where a lot of activity is involved, then your body will generate further free radicals. In order to protect your cells, joints and tissues, it is advisable to increase your intake of antioxidants to counteract this extra free radical activity.

Adequate rest and sleep is important in a weight loss program. While you are asleep, calcium and all the other minerals get to work. They are intimately linked to doing repair and renewal work within the body, like detoxifying the body as an example. These repair and renewal tasks are more difficult to do while you are awake and active.

This is why if you have a really late night (or several) or sleep irregular hours, you sometimes feel groggy in the morning, or irritable. This is your body giving you a message that it needs some time to sort some things out. It is important to listen to what your body is telling you. Ignore these messages at your peril.

Consult Your Doctor or a Naturopathic Doctor

With regard to how much of a particular product you may need to take, I have only included information for the Recommended Daily Allowance (RDA) for vitamins and minerals. I have not suggested any recommended amounts you should take of the featured herbal products, nor have I given any contra-indications.

In the body systems sections I have given you some product suggestions that have been used historically by herbalists and naturopaths, but no suggested dosage requirements.

The reason for this is that everyone is different. One person may need more of a particular product than the next person. Also, a particular product may suit one person, but not another.

Therefore I feel it is extremely important that you consult your doctor or a naturopathic doctor before commencing any supplement or herbal program, or changing your diet, or following any suggestions made in this book.

Additionally, you may be taking prescription medications for various health conditions which will, or could, have a negative impact on your health if you introduce vitamin or mineral supplements or an herbal program. Never take chances with your health.

I know that some doctors are not supportive of using a natural traditional route for health care. If your doctor feels this way and you would like to consider a more natural approach, then change your doctor and find one who is more supportive to your requirements.

Do You Live In a European Union Country

Of particular concern in Europe. In 2011 the European Union introduced the Herbal Medicines Directive which means the herbal industry has been all but destroyed by a draconian law which has all but banned the supply of herbal products within the European Union.

The excuse for issuing this directive is "to ensure public safety with regard to herbal products". I would have thought that something that has been used safely for hundreds (and in some cases thousands) of years would be safe for the public to take.

Many herbal products have been classified, not for use in food preparation (i.e. for cooking or garnishing purposes) but as "medicines" and a company now needs a license in order to sell them to the public. The cost of a license averages around $150,000 per herbal product. Yes, you read that correctly, $150,000 per herbal product.

Say you are a manufacturer and have just a small range of just 20 herbal products, that is going to cost you $3,000,000 in license fees, before you can sell anything. Very few manufacturers have that kind of money to waste on licenses for something that has been used safely for all those years.

All this new law is going to do is drive the supply of these safe, natural herbal products underground. With the power of modern communications and the Internet, all you have to do is spend a little time seeking out those herbal products you require from sources outside Europe. Many suppliers in other parts of the world—and especially the United States—will be more than happy to supply you, and will ship their products internationally. As the saying goes—where there's a will there's a way!!

About The Author

Brian B Jacques has been a natural health researcher for over thirty years. He has presented seminars worldwide on such diverse subjects as Health Related issues, Motivation and Personal Development. In addition he has written numerous eBooks, newsletters and articles on these subjects.

His very popular Series of Mini-Health Books includes:

- An Easy Way To Understand Eczema and Psoriasis
- An Easy Way To Understand Stress and Depression
- Amino Acids & Enzymes—What Are They & Why Do You Need Them
- An Easy Way To Understand Vitamins and Minerals
- An Easy Way To Understand Crohn's Disease and IBD
- An Easy Way To Understand Body Building For Men And Women
- An Easy Way To Understand Alzheimer's Disease
- An Easy Way To Understand Herpes
- An Easy Way To Understand Parkinson's Disease
- An Easy Way To Understand Autism
- An Easy Way To Understand Fibromyalgia
- The Little A–Z Dictionary of Herbal Remedies
- Effective Methods To Stop Smoking
- The Magic Of Vitamins & Minerals
- An Easy Way To Understand Your Body Systems
- An Easy Way To Understand Erectile Dysfunction
- An Easy Way To Understand Heart Disease, High Blood Pressure & Stroke
- An Easy Way To Understand Detoxing For Men & Women
- How To Lose Weight After 40
- How To Lose Weight And Maintain Your Ideal Weight Permanently

All these books are available as Kindle Editions (available from the Kindle Store on Amazon.com, and other countries Amazon sites where the Kindle platform is supported.) Many of these books are also available for the Barnes and Noble "Nook".In addition, all these titles will shortly be available as print editions from the Amazon website.

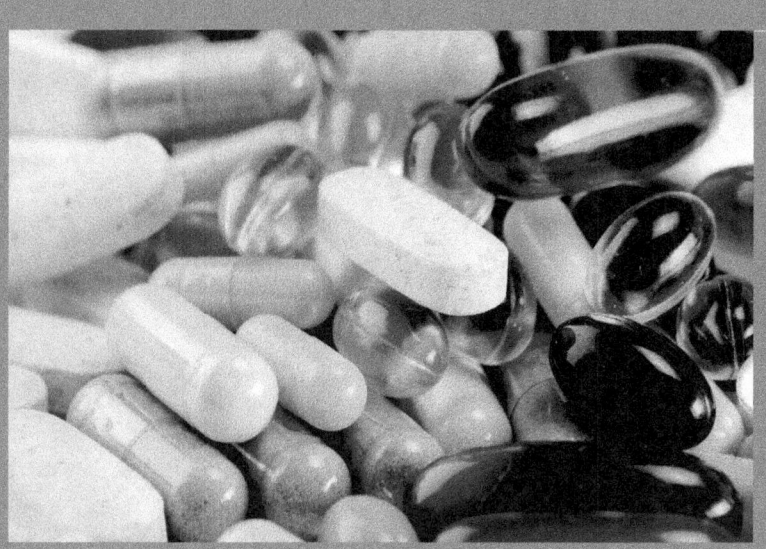

Index